How To Heal A Broken Leg – Fast!

I0407419

Understanding how to deal with a broken leg in order to start walking again quickly

"An overview of everything that will happen to you when you break your leg and how to handle it"

Dr. Jim Anderson

Published by:
Blue Elephant Consulting
Tampa, Florida

Printed in the United States of America

Library of Congress Control Number: 2016958088

ISBN-13: 978-1539756309
ISBN-10: 1539756300

Recent Books By The Author

Product Management

- What Product Managers Need To Know About World-Class Product Development: How Product Managers Can Create Successful Products

- How Product Managers Can Learn To Understand Their Customers: Techniques For Product Managers To Better Understand What Their Customers Really Want

Public Speaking

- Tools Speakers Need In Order To Give The Perfect Speech: What tools to use to create your next speech so that your message will be remembered forever!

- How To Create A Speech That Will Be Remembered

CIO Skills

- Becoming A Powerful And Effective Leader: Tips And Techniques That IT Managers Can Use In Order To Develop Leadership Skills

- CIO Secrets For Growing Innovation: Tips And Techniques For CIOs To Use In Order To Make Innovation Happen In Their IT Department

IT Manager Skills

- Save Yourself, Save Your Job – How To Manage Your IT Career: Secrets That IT Managers Can Use In Order To Have A Successful Career

- Growing Your CIO Career: How CIOs Can Work With The Entire Company In Order To Be Successful

Negotiating

- Learn How To Signal In Your Next Negotiation: How To Develop The Skill Of Effective Signaling In A Negotiation In Order To Get The Best Possible Outcome

- Learn The Skill Of Exploring In A Negotiation: How To Develop The Skill Of Exploring What Is Possible In A Negotiation In Order To Reach The Best Possible Deal

Note: See a complete list of books by Dr. Jim Anderson at the back of this book.

Acknowledgements

Any book like this one is the result of years of real-world work experience. In my over 25 years of working for 7 different firms, I have met countless fantastic people and I've been mentored by some truly exceptional ones. Although I've probably forgotten some of the people who made me the person that I am today, here is my attempt to finally give them the recognition that they so truly deserve:

- Thomas P. Anderson
- Art Puett
- Bobbi Marshall
- Bob Boggs

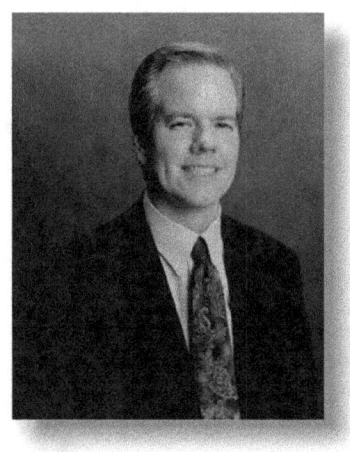

Dr. Jim Anderson

This book is dedicated to my wife Lori. None of this would have been possible without her love and support.

Thanks for the best years of my life (so far)...!

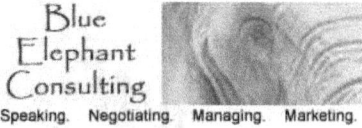

Blue Elephant Consulting

Speaking.   Negotiating.   Managing.   Marketing.

Table Of Contents

1	THE ACCIDENT	9
2	SURGERY	13
3	RECOVERING FROM SURGERY	17
3.1	Swelling	18
3.2	The Ice Machine	19
4	LIVING LIFE AFTER THE SURGERY	22
4.1	Leg Imobilizer	23
4.2	Crutches vs Wheelchair	25
4.3	Crutches	28
4.4	Crutch Maintenance	31
4.5	Showers	33
4.6	Cars / Driving	38
4.7	Sleeping	41
4.8	Eating Out	44
5	EXERCISING	47
5.1	Why Exercise?	49
5.2	Types Of Exercises That You Can Do	51
5.3	What You Can't Do	52
6	THE ROAD TO RECOVERY	54
6.1	What Happens While You Heal: The 90-Day Plan	55
6.2	Visits To the Doctor	56
6.3	Diet	59

6.4   Do More As Soon As You Can 63

6.5   Physical Therapy 64

6.6   Things You Can't Do 70

6.7   Sex...71

6.8   Emotional Issues 73

6.9   Urine 76

6.10   Walking Again 79

6.11   10 Months After The Accident..................................84

6.12   A Stretching Breakthrough.......................................86

7   THE LAST 15% 89

8   CONCLUSION 93

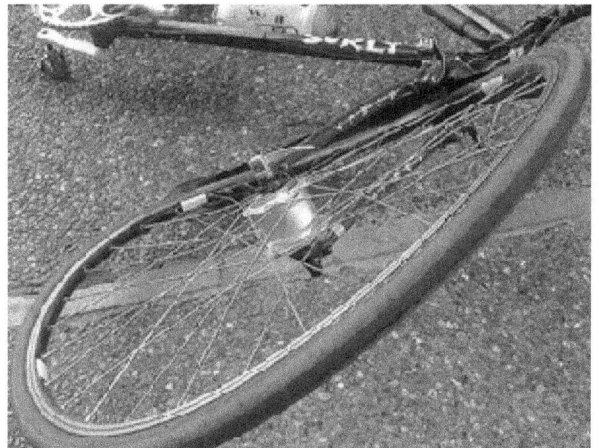

1   The Accident

First off, thank you very much for buying this book. Secondly, I'm very sorry that you have an interest in this topic. I suspect that either you or someone that you know has broken a bone. This is the kind of thing that seems to bedevil children but it turns out that it can strike any of us at any age.

I suspect that by this point in life you already know how to deal with having a cold, the flu, or a stomach ache. However, there is a very good chance that nobody ever told you how to deal with breaking a bone. That is exactly why this book was written. It turns out that your life is going to be turned upside down for a while and I want to make sure that you know what is coming and help you to prepare to deal with it.

Sadly, the reason that this book was written was because I broke my leg. It was a lovely summer day and I was out riding my bike around my neighborhood when the skies started to darken up and a light rain started to fall. Now one other thing that you have to know in order for this story to make sense is that the streets in my neighborhood had just been covered with a black "skim coat" to protect the asphalt and allow it to last longer.

What I didn't fully realize (although I had been warned about it by a neighbor) is that the newly sealed streets became quite slippery when they got wet. I went to turn my bike around in order to go home and avoid getting wet and the back wheel of my bike slide out from under me. Down I went right there in the middle of the road. I don't really remember falling (I was wearing a helmet and so that was a good thing), but what I did instantly know was that there was something seriously wrong with my left leg.

All that I knew was that I was not going to be able to stand up on that leg. As the rain picked up in intensity I fumbled for my cell phone to call my wife at home come pick me up. Of course this was the one time that my cell phone decided that it didn't want to stop playing the music that I had just been listening to. Somehow I finally get the phone part of the phone to work and was able to tell my wife "come pick me up, I've fallen and it's bad".

Thankfully our relationship is strong enough that she showed up in just a couple of minutes. While she pushed my bike to the side of the road, I dragged myself into the back of the minivan and we were off to the hospital.

At this point in time I was in discomfort, but not what I would really call pain. Clearly there was something wrong with my leg, but I had no idea what it was: torn ligaments, a really bad bruise? At the hospital they took pictures and the young doctor who was on staff that evening told me that I had fractured my Tibula.

Just in case your knowledge of human anatomy is not as good as it should be, the Tibula is the big bone in the bottom part of your leg right by your calf. It forms sort of a "cup" that your thigh bone fits into and that's how the two parts of your leg work together to allow you to bend your leg, walk, and run. The doctor was rather coy about how I was going to get this problem fixed outside of saying that I needed to see an orthopedic surgeon. I pressed him for some details on what was going to have to be done to fix me up and he finally said the "S" word — surgery.

At the hospital they provided me with what would soon become my constant companions: a leg immobilizer and crutches. The leg immobilizer consisted of a foam pad that is about three feet by two feet in dimensions. It has three pieces of metal that can be slid into it in order to prevent the knee from moving backwards or to either side. It comes with six pieces of Velcro that are used to secure it to the leg.

My leg was wrapped in an Ace bandage because the skin had gotten pretty beat up when I fell off the bike. This meant my wrapped leg was now immobilized. I am six and half feet tall — very tall. The crutches that they provided me with would have only been able to be extend one more position. I'm not sure what they would have done then! I quickly learned how to maneuver myself around on the crutches as we left the hospital.

When you discover that you are going to need major medical work done on you, there is a period of shock and adjustment that is necessary. I will confess that I still harbored a deep hope that perhaps the X-rays that they had taken at the hospital were wrong. Maybe between the time that I first went to the hospital and when I would finally see my orthopedic surgeon I just might heal up all by myself. I mean, if it was just a little nick to the bone, I could probably drink some milk, stay off the leg, and things would be considerably better the next time that a doctor took a look at me. Right?

As you may have guessed by now, my hopes were quickly dashed when a week later I finally had a chance to meet the orthopedic surgeon. He's a great guy and a fine surgeon, but man does his bedside manner leave something to be desired! He gave it to me straight: you are a humpty dumpy. I had fallen off of the proverbial wall and had basically shattered my Tibula.

It turns out that I had also broken the top of the smaller bone that lives in the lower part of your leg also. However, the good doctor was not too concerned by this — it would heal on its own given time. The bigger question was how were we going to put the 3-4 pieces that my Tibula had shattered into back together again? It turns out that the doctor had an answer to this: a plate and potentially up to 12 screws. I did not like that option one bit. However, I was not in the driver's seat on this one and so I said "thanks" and we scheduled my surgery for one week in the future.

You know that I had to ask him: how long is it going to take me to recover. How long until I'll be able to walk normally again? I didn't like his answer at all. He said that it was going to take me three months to recover from just the surgery. He said that in order to regain full use of my broken leg and be back to the way that things were before the break in some cases takes up to a full year. Right then and there I vowed that this would not be me. I was going to back to normal as soon as humanly possible!

Just to be clear — I had a broken leg. So for the time that separated my visit to the hospital to when I had my surgery, I was on my own. A total of 8 days passed from when I broke my leg to when I had surgery. Not a lot of time by normal standards; however, it's a very long time when all of a sudden you discover that you can't do most of the things that you normally do!

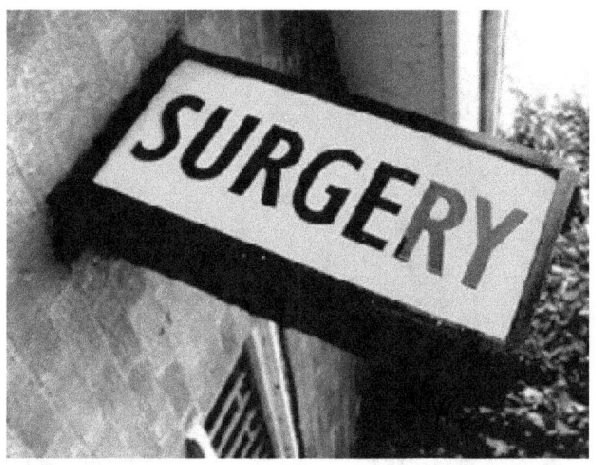

2   Surgery

So let me state this up front: I don't really like hospitals. The thought of me having to go to one, be operated on, and then recover there filled me with dread. Since I had shattered my Tibula I required surgery. If you've simply broken a bone into two parts, you may be able to get away with having the pieces fitted together and then having a cast placed on them. If this is your situation, then congratulations — it could have been much worse. My case was a bit more serious.

In talking with my orthopedic surgeon he revealed to me that what I had done to myself is called a "Tibial Plateau Fracture". Basically I had broken the top part of the big bone in my lower left leg off. This is a tricky break to fix because of where the screws that will hold the bones back together need to be placed.

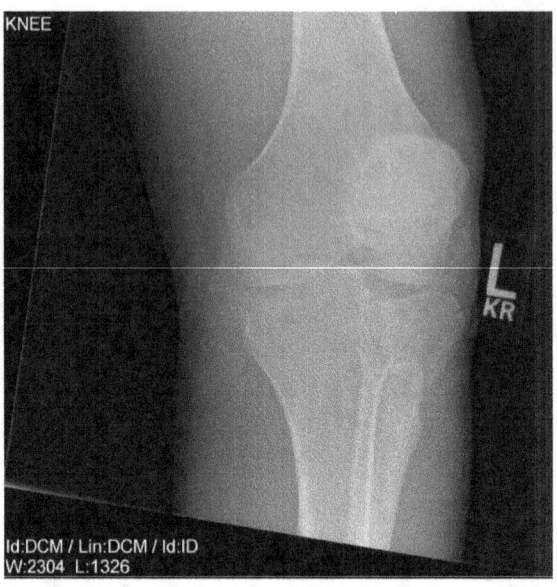

Figure 1: An X-Ray of the author's broken Tibula

My surgery was going to take upwards of about four hours. During the surgery he was going to be inserting a roughly 5" metal plate into my leg and then securing it to the bones that had shattered using screws. I was amazed to discover that this was considered to be outpatient surgery — I was eligible to go home that evening.

My surgeon cautioned me against doing that. What he told me was that when I went home, he would be prescribing a routine pain killer. However, I would be experiencing my most significant discomfort after the painkillers that they had given me for surgery wore off — about four hours after the whole thing was done. He pointed out to me that if I chose to stay in the hospital overnight I would have access to more powerful pain killers (morphine) and that might make things go a bit smoother for me on that first night.

On the day of the surgery, I showed up at the hospital and was escorted back to a room to get ready for surgery. I stripped down to my undies and handed all of my clothes and my crutches to my wife for safekeeping. All of the normal prep work was done: my temperature was taken, my blood pressure was checked, and they started an IV drip.

I'd like to be able to tell you something about the surgery itself, but the hospital staff played a cruel trick on me. Perhaps I had been a bit too verbose with them, but as the time approached for me to be wheeled down to the operating room they gave me what they called "an anxiety relaxer" which to me sounded like something that would calm me down. I was wrong, as I was being wheeled down the hall I went unconscious and didn't wake up until the surgery was over and done with.

As I came to in my hospital room, I did not feel any pain. That was probably due to the surgery pain killers that were still in my system. My knee was now wrapped in an ACE bandage and it did throb a bit. There are really only two key points to my post-operative hospital stay that you may be interested in: urination and pain killers.

I am a male and since walking at this stage of the game was not an option because I probably would have been too woozy due to my medications, I was provided with a clear plastic jug that had a bent neck to it. This was what I was to urinate into when I had to go. During the day it was not a problem because I had not really drunk very much during the day; however, I did a good job of filling it at night.

While I was in the hospital, my pain and discomfort was managed by providing me with morphine. I was given a button that I could push whenever I felt discomfort. There was a green light on a machine. When the green light was on, I could press the button. When I did this the green light went off and stayed off for about 15 minutes.

I believe that each time I pressed the green button I then got a shot of morphine. As I slept that night I would wake up every so often. I quickly learned that if I saw the green light on, I needed to push my button no matter how my knee felt — it was going to feel worse later on if I didn't. Sometime in the morning after I had woken up, I used up the last of the morphine just before the hospital staff would have cut me off anyway. As they took the machine away I discovered that I had pushed the button 30 times over the course of the night.

Leaving the hospital was relatively uneventful. I had to get out of bed and using my crutches I had to show a nurse that I could make it up and down a hall by myself. Once she was convinced that I could do this, she called for a wheelchair and I was taken to the curb where once again I crawled into my minivan and was taken home.

The doctor's orders were very, very clear. Unless I wanted to come back to him for a full knee replacement I was to not put any weight on my broken leg. This was going to be my life for the next 90 days (that's three months).

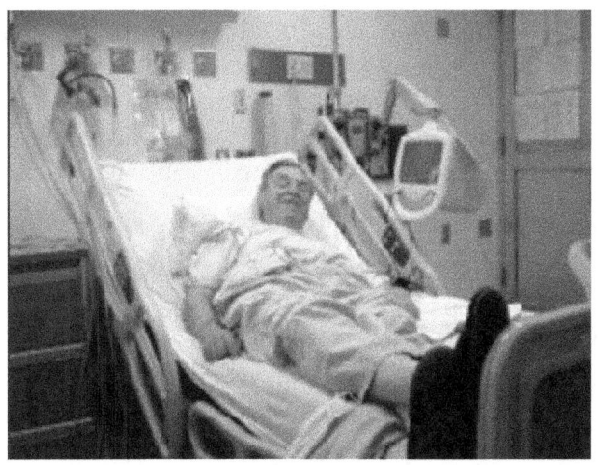

3   Recovering From Surgery

If you've just broken a bone and not fractured it, your recovery may be a bit different than mine was. Since I had fractured my Tibula, what the doctor had to do was to make a "reverse 7" cut just below my left knee and then trailing down my left leg. All in all, the cut was roughly 3" x 5". The longer part of the cut was required because the doctor had to insert a plate and then secure it to my leg bone with the help of seven screws. The screws extended through various pieces of my fractured Tibula and served to pull the pieces back into place.

What's interesting is that apparently the screws came with guide wires to assist in getting them into place and my doctor had some difficulties removing all of the guide wires and so he ended up having to make another incision on the back of my knee just to get to the wires. When this operation was done, multiple levels of stitches were then used to seal the wound up and 18 staples were used on the outside of the wound to hold it closed. The entire area was covered in gauze and then wrapped in an ACE bandage.

One of the first challenges that I encountered with my wound was showers. Clearly the ACE bandage and the gauze had to come off, but was it ok to expose the wound to rushing shower water? In the end my wife and decided to compromise. What I did in the early days was to drape a washcloth over the wound while I was in the shower just to prevent the rushing water from flowing over it and perhaps causing the wound to open.

Over time the wound appeared to be healing well. On my third follow-up trip to the doctor he announced that my metal staples could be removed. As you might imagine, this was not a comfortable process. The medical assistant who actually did the removal used a numbing spray to desensitize the area where she would be removing the staples before she pulled them out. However, she would often exceed the area where she had sprayed and that didn't feel good. By the way, 18 staples is a lot of staples and it took a good 5 minutes to remove them all.

Over the next week or so, my wife noticed a disturbing sequence of events. My wound was starting to open up. We were concerned enough about this to schedule an unplanned meeting with the doctor to have him take a look at it. When he saw what was happening he announced that I was having a reaction to the four layers of stitches that had been used to seal up the wound.

He prescribed an antibiotic that I then took for the next 15 days, twice a day. During this time my wife would treat the open wound with a sterilization solution and then pat it dry. Over time the wound started to close up again and by the time that I completed the round of antibiotics, the wound was completely sealed.

3.1   Swelling

As you may well imagine, if your breakage requires you to have surgery, that's going to be a fairly traumatic event for your body. Nobody (pun intended) likes to be cut open, perhaps have a metal plate or rod inserted, have a few screws put in place and then be sewn up again. In my case, when I shattered my Tibula my surgery required that I have a 5" plate placed in my leg which was then secured in place by 7 screws.

Once this had been accomplished, the doctors used four layers of stitches to close up the hole that they had created. Afterwards my doctor told me that because the plate had been inserted so close to the knee, there was not a lot of extra skin and such to work with so they had some challenges closing up the wound.

Your greatest period of discomfort will occur, naturally, after the surgery. Your body has been traumatized and it's going to let you know that it's not happy about what has just happened. Your #1 goal at this point in time is going to be to keep the site of the surgery packed in ice.

The ice will help to reduce the swelling that will be occurring. Hopefully it goes without saying, but I'll say it once again: whenever you are dealing with something cold, you don't want to have it touch your skin. If you do, then there is a very good chance that you may end up getting frostbite and that will just make a bad situation even worse.

Obviously keeping a part of the body packed in ice involves getting some of those ice packs that you can toss into the freezer, freezing them, and then placing them on the other side of a towel that you've placed on you broken bone. However, you can well imagine how tedious this is going to become over the one to two weeks that you'll be needing the ice.

3.2   The Ice Machine

Those ice packs melt and they will have to be replaced with fresh ice packs. You can't move easily and so this is quickly going to become yet another burden on your care giver.

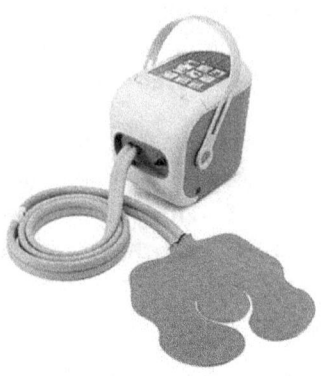

Figure 2: Ossur Cold Rush - Cold Therapy System

In my case we got lucky. My wife had been talking with a friend whose husband had injured himself awhile back and she happened to remark that they had purchased a machine that circulated ice water through a pad that was placed on the injured area. Ice water was placed in the machine and this meant that it stayed cold for a longer time than individual ice packs and it delivered a colder experience also.

This caught our attention. My wife went on to Amazon and discovered the Ossur Cold Rush Compact Cold Therapy System (http://amzn.to/1kJoJHm). The cost of this system was $134, but my wife was able to get one cheaper on Craig's List.

This system worked like a charm for me. I would always place a dish towel on my leg first and then I would place the cooling pad on top of that. The cooling pad would get very cold very quickly and so it was important that it never touch skin. The manufacture recommends not using their product at night and that's probably a good idea. However, I wanted to sleep well and I figured that if I could keep my broken leg cool during the night I might be able to fall asleep faster so I did use it at night.

As you might well imagine, trying to keep a cooling pad in place while tossing and turning at night was a bit of a challenge. I ended up wrapping the pad in a towel and basically securing it to my leg. It would fall off sometimes, but I feel that it helped me to ignore my leg more and fall asleep faster.

In the end, by keeping my leg cold for a significant amount of the time after surgery I believe that I successfully avoided a lot of the problems that people have when their body reacts to the events of the surgery. I did have some swelling, but nothing of any real significance.

By using the Ossur system at night, I was not as distracted by my sore leg and I felt as though I was able to fall asleep faster than I would have been able to without it. All in all, I keep my leg packed in ice for about three weeks. After that point in time, I felt that the possibility of swelling had passed and the hassle of keeping the machine filled with ice water was no longer worth it for me.

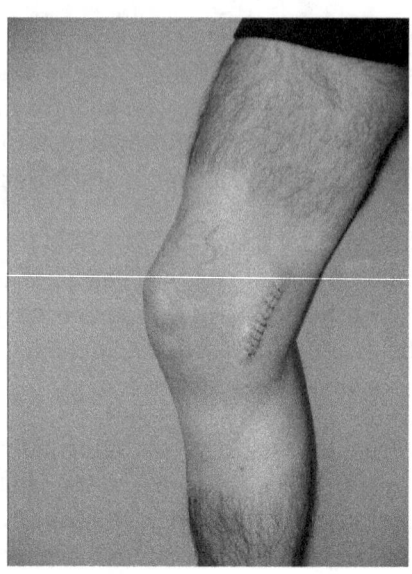

4   Living Life After The Surgery

Just imagine if you were a professional sports player. You'd only be valuable to your team when you were on the field and so if you broke your leg, the team would want to do everything in their power to get you healed up and back on that field as soon as possible. Now, they wouldn't have any magic fairy dust that they could sprinkle on you to hurry things up, but they could put a team of doctors and massage therapists at your beck and call. How fantastic would that be? I'm pretty sure that they could get your leg to do what it's supposed to do as fast as possible. The problem here, of course, is that you are NOT a professional sports figure.

What this means for you is that your recovery after your surgery is going to be in your hands. Nobody else's. Your family and friends who have been so supportive so far, are going to be getting a little tired of having to do things for you. You need to realize this and start to both take on more tasks and start to plan how you are going to manage your recovery.

Life after the surgery for me was very similar to life before the surgery, but there was just a lot more to it. Now that I had had my broken bone repaired I found myself needing my leg immobilizer much more because I didn't want to somehow step wrong or fall over and once again screw up my already broken leg. During your recovery time, your life is going to be more complicated and you are going to have to make adjustments to accomplish things that you used to be able to do without thinking about them.

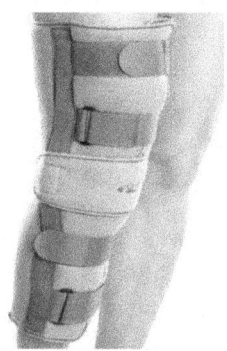

4.1   Leg Imobilizer

The evening that I went to the hospital with my broken leg, I received a gift that would stay with me for the next two months. The hospital staff gave me what they called a "leg immobilizer" to wear home. This consists of a 3' x 2' piece of spongy fabric that had long vertical pockets into which could be slide three metal bars.

It wrapped around my knee with the assistance of 6 long Velcro straps. While I was wearing this contraption, my leg was held straight and I could not bend it. The thinking is that if I was to stumble or fall, the leg immobilizer would protect my broken bones and would prevent them from being forcibly twisted to either side.

I wore the leg immobilizer for two months straight. I would not wear it to bed and I, perhaps obviously, did not wear it when I was taking a shower. Something interesting about this. When I removed the immobilizer and headed to the shower, I felt incredibly exposed. I realized that both this journey and my time in the shower were arguably the most dangerous times of the day as far as further injuring my break went. It was with a real sense of relief that I was able to once again put the immobilizer on after a shower.

As you might imagine, any piece of clothing that you wear daily will start to take some wear and tear. In my case, the parts of the fabric that the Velcro straps would attach to started to show some real wear. I was lucky and somehow avoided getting any food or other stains on the fabric during my time wearing it. My wife did mention after about a month that she believed that it had developed its own unique odor.

This problem was solved on Friday nights. Upon taking the immobilizer off to go to bed, I would Febreze the front and the back. It would then have overnight to dry out and in the morning it would have a fresh clean smell — it was ready for another week of constant wearing.

I did not have any problems with the immobilizer rubbing against my wound. The reason for this was because since I had had surgery, my wound was covered by an ACE bandage. Any rubbing that did occur was between the immobilizer and my ACE bandage.

Clothes were a bit of a problem when I was wearing the immobilizer. When it was in place, there was no way that pants could be fit over it. The immobilizer coupled with my leg's post-surgery swelling and the ACE bandage made quite a large package.

I have the benefit of living in Florida in the U.S.A. What this means is that the outside temperature is almost always very comfortable. I was able to deal with my wardrobe situation by switching from business clothes to shorts for the duration of my recovery. I would slide both underwear and shorts on in the morning before putting the immobilizer on and then in the evening I would take the immobilizer off before getting undressed.

I would wear the immobilizer for the entire day with one exception. During lunch I would undo the Velcro straps and free my leg. While it was freed, I would perform my leg exercises. Once these were over and done with, I would take the time to seal up each of the six Velcro straps and I would be on my way once again.

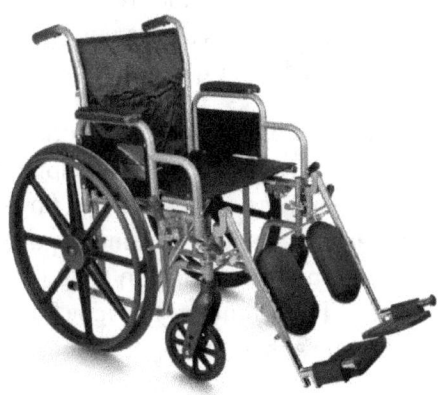

4.2 Crutches vs Wheelchair

Depending on how badly you've hurt yourself, you are going to be facing a big question. No matter if you are wearing a cast or if you've had to go the surgery route, your mobility for the near term future is going to depend on you getting some help from a mechanical device. What this means is that you are going to have to choose between crutches or a wheelchair.

I must confess that I was both lucky and torn. I had a friend whose elderly father had just been moved into a nursing home and so the two wheelchairs that they had been using to transport him when he was living with them were just sitting around. My friend was kind enough to bring both chairs over to my house when he heard about my leg. The hospital had provided me with a new set of crutches and then my wife remembered that from a long-ago leg incident that I had had with my other knee, we already owned a fine pair of crutches. What this all meant is that I was handicap transportation wealthy. Now I just needed to decide which method I wanted to use.

Let's face it: although perhaps none of us want to find ourselves in a wheelchair, they are pretty cool to look at. Plus the thought of not having to stand and being able to just wheel ourselves around everywhere and then having a chair waiting for us when we got there was a pretty powerful pull towards adopting the wheelchair as my primary mode of transportation.

In the spirit of openness I must confess that I even went so far as to go on the Amazon online shopping site in order to locate and purchase some gloves without finger tips that I had seen other people in wheelchairs using to get around. It turns out that since your hand is coming in contact with the wheel as you propel yourself and you don't exactly know where that wheel has been, the gloves are a good idea.

My initial interest in using the wheelchairs that I had been loaned quickly started to fade away. What happened is that I started to realize that it was going to be a big inconvenience. In order to get out of the house, I had suggested to my wife that she push me around the neighborhood at night.

Soon I wanted to be the one who was propelling myself, not her. Very quickly I discovered that it is hard to propel a wheelchair in a straight line. Any slight curvature in the road or path that you are on will send you off in a given direction. Additionally, if you don't perfectly match your right and left hand pushes on the wheel, then you'll be sending yourself off to one side or the other.

Another problem that the wheelchair presented was that it was quite cumbersome and heavy. Wheelchairs do collapse so that they can be stowed and transported, but they are very heavy. In my situation, I had to imagine that I had driven somewhere, got out of my car and somehow had made it back to the trunk of the car, opened the trunk, and then managed standing on one leg to lift the heavy wheelchair out of the trunk and open it up so that I could sit in it. There was no way that I was going to be able to do all of that.

As you can well imagine by now, I went with the crutches. The two wheelchairs lay abandoned in my house now only occasionally played with by my children and their friends.

The crutches do require more effort on my part to get around, but they have a number of clear advantages. I can get very carefully get into narrow spaces. I can actually move quite quickly when I'm moving in a straight line and I get some rhythm going. Crutches also allow you to pivot 180 degrees very easily. However, one big difference between crutches and a wheelchair is that you can't carry anything in your hands when you are using crutches whereas you can place things in your lap when you are using a wheelchair.

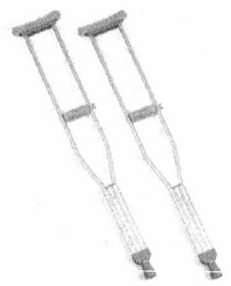

4.3   Crutches

So let's talk about crutches, shall we? In my case, crutches became how I got around for just a bit over three months. One thing that I realized when I was finally able to get off of using crutches was that I had become very adept at using the crutches. I could move around quite quickly and cover a great deal of ground. I can't say that this will happen for everyone, but it sure did happen for me.

One of the most important things that you need to realize about using crutches is how to properly use them. Specifically, don't use them wrong! What I mean by this is that I've seen a lot of people on crutches with big fancy pillows attached to the part of the crutch that goes under their arms. Clearly they were using the crutches incorrectly.

What I mean by this is that holding on to the crutches and moving on the crutches needs to all be done by your wrists and forearms. Your armpits are not involved in this process at all. The only thing that your armpits should be doing is allowing you to keep your crutches steady and not rotating either forward or backwards. You should be squeezing the sides of your crutches with your armpits and not resting on them. At the end of the day, your armpits should not be sore from using crutches!

One of the biggest challenges that you'll face when you are on crutches is stairs. There are many different ways to handle stairs and you are going to have to pick the one that you feel works the best for you. In my case, the stairs that I encountered the most were the ones in my house. I slept and ate on the first floor, my office was located on the second floor. In the early days of using crutches, I would walk up the stairs using my crutches.

Now, you may already be trying to picture this in your head and you'd be correct — this was a risky move. I would place the crutch ends on the next step up, move my "bad" foot to hover over that step, and then lift up with my good foot and the crutches at the same time in order to move my good foot to the next stair. There was an element of risk to this maneuver.

While I was moving up to the next step, I could possibly lose my balance and fall if I was not careful. This never happened to me and I don't think that I even came close, but I was always aware of the possibility. I tried to minimize the chances of something bad happening by leaning forward so that if I did fall, I would at least fall forwards rather than backwards down the stairs.

Eventually, I decided that since I was going up and down these stairs so much, the risk associated with navigating them while on crutches was too much. I changed my stair climbing approach. I would approach the stairs at the bottom, rest my crutches on the stairs, sit down on the bottom stair with my feet resting on a stair below me and then proceed to use my wrists and forearms to boost my butt up the stairs one stair at a time.

I would have to stop occasionally and throw my crutches up the stairs in front of me every so often. At the top of the stairs I had positioned a chair and I would back into it and then use my arms to boost my bottom up and end up sitting on the chair. Once I was there, I could pick up my crutches and make my way across the room. Going down the stairs simply meant reversing this process.

I must confess that I got lucky. I was able to further optimize my stair climbing strategy in my house. My wife discovered that we owned another set of crutches that I must have used back when I had my other knee operated on. We ended up putting these crutches upstairs. What this meant was that I could now come to the bottom of the stairs, place my crutches against the wall and then proceed to haul myself up the stairs without having to go to the effort of bringing my crutches along. Truly I was living in the lap of luxury.

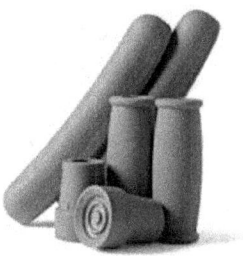

4.4   Crutch Maintenance

Just in case you had not already realized it, three months (90 days) is a long time to use a single set of crutches. You need to realize that a crutch consists of three parts that can wear out over time: the rubber bottom stopper, the hand grips, and the armpit cushions. Over time and constant usage, your crutches are going to wear out.

You'll see the wear show up in different places: the rubber grips that your hands hold on to will start to fail first — they'll start to become looser and will start to rotate. The rubber tips at the bottom of the crutches will also wear out. Eventually the aluminum shaft will poke through the rubber tip from the top. The pieces of rubber at the top of the crutches will also start to wear; however, if you are using your crutches correctly, this is where you'll have the least amount of wear.

The good news here is that a replacement kit with everything that you'll need is available from Amazon for roughly US$12. Here's the link: http://amzn.to/1QxljVj

One thing that happened with my crutches that caught me by surprise is that the top pieces had a tendency to fall off. When this happened once and I had to hobble around for a bit searching for the missing pad, I discovered how uncomfortable it was to use crutches with a hard piece of plastic at the top of the crutch.

Once I realized this I vowed to make sure that my top parts never accidentally fell off again. My first attempt to solve this problem consisted of using Velcro to secure the pad to the crutch. It turns out that this did not work out so well — the two pieces of Velcro joined together and pulled away from the surfaces that they were attached to thus not securing anything in place.

Once I had realized that this had failed, I then upped my game and used industrial cement to glue the top part in place. This probably means that I could not easily replace the top pads, but that was ok because they didn't seem to be wearing very much since I was using my crutches properly and not putting much weight on the top cushions.

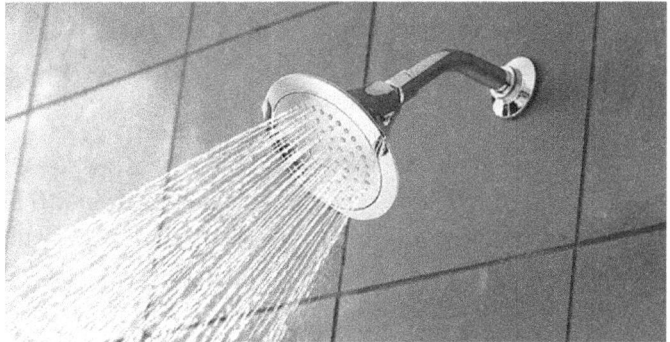

4.5 Showers

In my humble opinion, taking a shower when you have a broken leg is the single most dangerous thing that you'll do. The possibility of slipping and falling when you don't have full control over both of your legs is a real danger. It's because of this fact that whenever I got ready to take a shower I would repeat my mantra "safety first". Immediately after my surgery, I really was not up to taking a shower.

It was during this time that my wife and I made the grand discovery that a modern human male can go for about four days without showering before he starts to smell like he's spent the weekend out camping with the boys. When it did become time for me to take a shower in the beginning, it was a major production. I would have to sit on the bed and strip down.

Meanwhile, my wife would run the shower water in order to get it warm enough. Once she had accomplished this, she would call me into the bathroom. Once I arrived, she would assist me in getting into the shower. Once in, I would sit on the shelf that our shower has in the back. My wife would then place a washcloth over my surgery wound (we were not sure if it really should be exposed to running water at this stage of the game) and then she would turn the shower back on and point it at my head. I would spend the next five minutes or so washing my hair and soaping myself up. Once I was done, I'd call out for her to come back. She'd turn the water off, hand me a towel, and then help me get out of the shower.

You can well imagine how eager I was to try to become more independent when it came to taking showers. The level of assistance that I was requiring was making me feel as though I was a very old man. Over time was I was able to become more independent. Safety was always my first concern. Upon entering the bathroom on my crutches I would position a rug in front of the shower door so that my crutches would not slip if there was any water there.

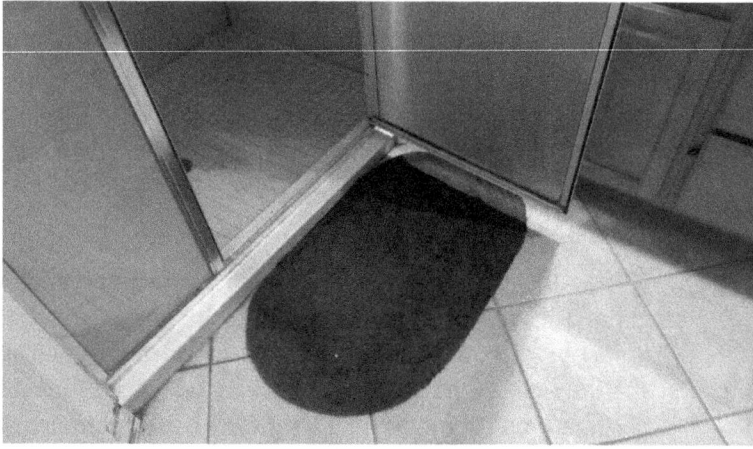

Figure 3: Larger rug outside of shower

Next, I would get a smaller rug and manually position it inside of the shower so that when I stepped into the shower on my crutches I would not slip.

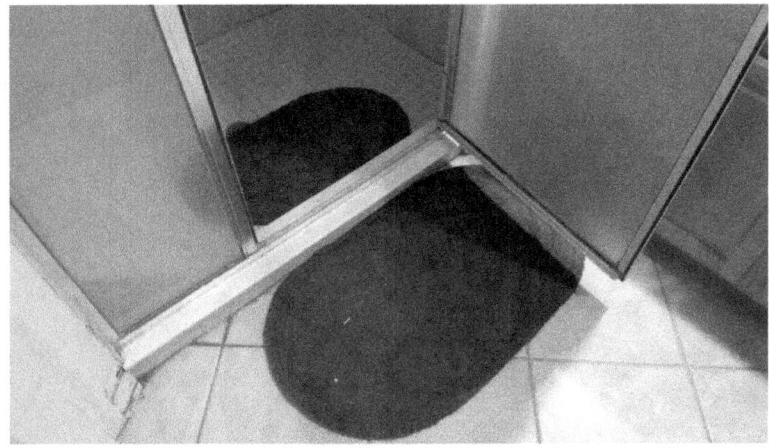

Figure 4: Two rugs for shower - one inside and one outside

The process for gaining access to the shower consisted of my lining my crutches up at the door to the shower, standing on my good foot, placing the ends of both crutches into the shower and then maneuvering my broken leg over the doorway into the shower and then using the crutches to boost my good leg up and over the doorway into the shower.

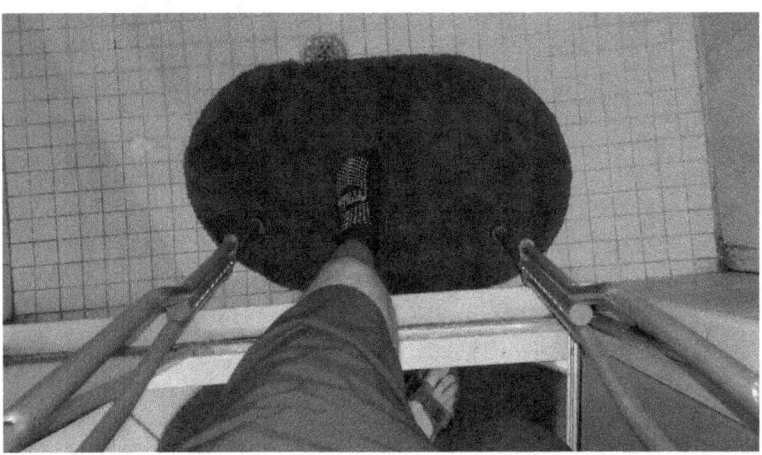

Figure 5: Stepping into the shower onto small rug

Once in the shower I would spin around on my crutches to get off of the rug that I was on. I would then drape it over the shower door so that I could get to it later on and finally I would place both crutches outside of the shower.

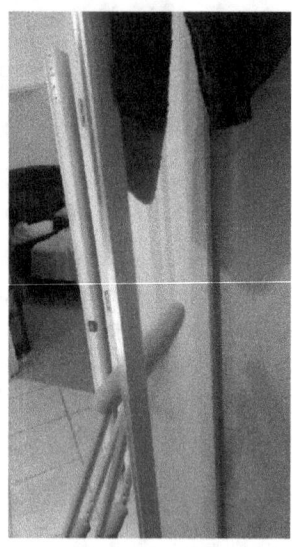

Figure 6: Crutches stored outside of shower during shower

Taking the shower was relatively easy; however, I found that I really could not move. I was also positioned off to one side (in my case close to the door). This meant that I had to reposition the shower head to point at me. The problem with this is that sometimes I would forget to reposition the shower head once I was done with my shower and on more than one occasion family members reported being soaked as they turned the shower on because I had left the shower head pointed towards them.

My biggest shower challenge was washing my backside since I could not easily turn around in the shower. What I eventually discovered was that if I faced the shower head and ducked my head down and let the water run down my back, it was the same as if I had been able to turn around.

Getting out of the shower was very much the same as getting into the shower, just done in reverse. I would reach up and get down the small rug that I had used in the shower when getting in. I would once again place it on the floor in the shower and then stand on it using my crutches. Getting out of the shower required me to position the ends of both of my crutches outside of the shower on the larger rug that was there, position my broken foot outside of the shower, and then boost my good foot outside the shower using the crutches.

Although taking a shower was still a major effort, it was a major effort only for me. I was able to do it without any assistance from my wife and that was a great feeling considering everything else that I was not currently able to do by myself.

I will confess that I was so nervous about falling and hurting myself while taking a shower that just prior to getting into the shower I would go into the bedroom and make sure that all of the doors between where I was and where my wife currently was were open. I figured that should I fall, by having the doors open she would more easily be able to hear my pitiful cries for help. Thankfully it never came to this!

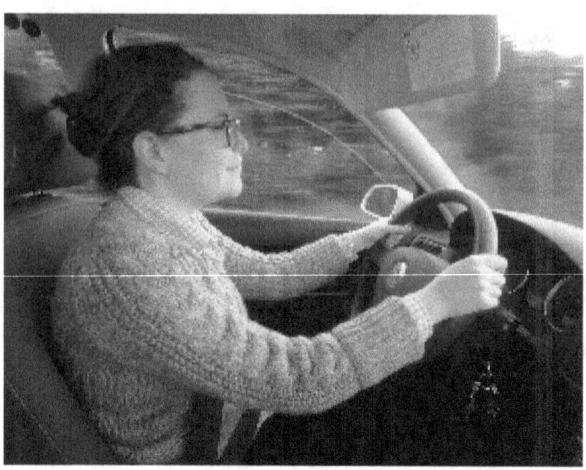

4.6 Cars / Driving

A side effect of breaking your leg is that all of a sudden your world becomes a lot smaller. What this means is that because it is now hard to get around, you don't. You set up your house to accommodate your new limited mobility. The things that you need are placed where you can get them and you establish "places that you go" such as in front of the TV or at the dining table and your day pretty much consists of traveling between those spots. All of this new domestic living does bring up an interesting question: what about cars and driving?

A lot of this is going to have to do with a couple of key issues. The first, of course, is what did you break? If it is your right leg, you've got a big problem because our cars are set up to have us drive them using our right leg. If it's your left leg, then you are in a much better position — the left leg really does not do that much when you are driving and so you should be able to do all of the things that you normally do. In the case of a broken left leg your biggest issue will be trying to fit yourself into the driver's seat.

The second big issue is what type of car you drive. If you drive an automatic transmission that allows you to drive using just one leg, then you are in a good place. If you drive a manual transmission then things are going to get a bit trickery — they require two feet and you may or may not be able to accomplish this. Some investigation on your part is going to be required.

First off, let me state that if there are any challenges to you driving, then don't do it. Have someone else drive you where you need to go and be done with it. However, if you are of the mind that you want to investigate driving yourself, then let's continue our discussion.

If you have broken you right leg, you have some significant challenges ahead of you. The first of these is that with a cast or a leg immobilizer you are not going to be able to bend your leg and move between the gas and break petals like you used to. You can investigate using your left leg to accomplish these tasks. The good news is that it can be done, the bad news is that it will feel very strange indeed.

I have no experience trying to drive a car using my left foot and so you are going to have to do some very careful experimentation to see if this is even an option for you. Let me once again state that let me state that if there are any challenges to you driving, then don't do it. Have someone else drive you where you need to go — safety first.

If you've broken your left leg, you are in a much better situation. Your biggest challenge here is going to be getting into the car. Since your broken leg is probably immobilized via a brace or a cast, your left leg will not be bending that much. This means that you'll have to sit back as far as your extended left leg requires you to sit.

This may be a bit of a problem when it comes to reaching the gas and break petal with your right foot. One technique that I found to be helpful was that I discovered that I could extend my left foot further underneath the dashboard by stretching it past the break petal on its left hand side. This didn't buy me that much more room, perhaps only a couple of inches, but in my case that was all that I needed to feel more comfortable.

If you are able to work out the whole feet and driving thing, you are still going to be facing the challenge of what to do with your crutches while driving (assuming that you've gone the crutch route). In my case I was driving a 2009 Honda Accord and with a little investigation I discovered that the back seat had a pull down armrest in the middle of the back bench seat. In the opening that this created in the back seat cushion there was a small door.

When this door was opened, a pass-through to the trunk no bigger than 4" x 6" was created. I opened this door and upon getting into the car would maneuver the crutches so that the tips would pass through this opening and into the trunk. In this manner I was able to secure my crutches and not have them roll around while I was driving.

I almost hate to bring this up, but in the eyes of the law you are now officially handicapped. You may not like having that label applied to you, but now is the time to make the most of it. In terms of driving what this means is that you are probably eligible to receive a temporary handicapped placard to hand from your rear view mirror.

The way that you go about getting one of these is to have your doctor provide you with proof of need and then you take this to your local department of motor vehicles to get the placard. This will allow you to park in all of those handicapped spots that you've always driven by in the past.

I was not all that happy about now fitting this description; however, when I was using crutches it was a big advantage to be able to park up close to the businesses that I was visiting. These placards are generally only good for about 6 months so you'll probably only need to get one.

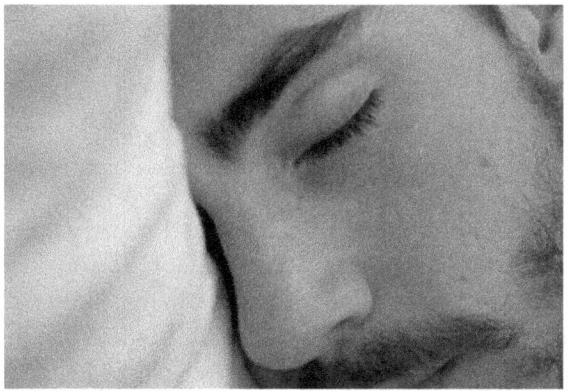

4.7 Sleeping

When you break your leg, all of a sudden sleeping becomes a very big deal. You really just want the time to pass quickly until you are all healed and you view the more time that you spend sleeping as progress towards this goal. However, as with all such things in life, there are some challenges here. Specifically your leg hurts both from being broken in the first place and then from any surgery that you've had done on it. Finding the right way to sleep can be quite a challenge.

The first thing that you are going to want to do is to set yourself up to get a good night's sleep. You probably already know this drill: don't drink any stimulants before going to bed, try to relax, etc. In my case, one day I had a large soda a couple of hours before going to bed and I was up all night. I couldn't figure out what I had done wrong until I realized that having the soda was not a good idea, but the fact that I was not moving around all that much meant that I had not been able to burn the soda off before going to bed and that's why it had hit me so hard.

Once you are in bed, you are going to want to find the right position to sleep in. I'm here to tell you that you have roughly three positions to choose from: pointing to the left, sleeping on your back, and pointing to the right. In my case, since I had effectively damaged my left knee bending my left leg was a real challenge. What I discovered was that when I was sleeping pointing to left my left knee didn't like having any pressure from the right knee placed on it. I was able to partially solve this problem by sleeping with a pillow between my knees.

This actually brings up a very good point: when you have a broken leg, pillows are your friend. I truly don't think that you can ever have enough of them. In my case, my left leg physically hurt me if I stretched it out. At this point in time, I don't think that it was the bones that were causing me problems, it was the simple fact that I had not been walking on this leg and the muscles and such were starting to atrophy and shrink up.

The position that felt best for my broken leg was for me to be on my back and the left leg slightly bent so that it was not stretched out. The way that I was able to make this happen was by placing a pillow under my left knee and resting the leg on it. Because of who I am, I tried to get away from relying on this to go to sleep as soon as possible; however, I am more than willing to admit that if I was having a bad night, I'd pull that extra pillow into bed, prop up my knee and I'd be asleep shortly thereafter.

Sleeping on your back has never been something that I have found to be very comfortable. However, when you have a broken leg and you are trying to find a way to fall asleep, you will try almost anything. This meant that I gave "back sleeping" a try.

What's interesting about this position is that in order to get comfortable, you really need to extend both of your legs. In my case, the left leg really didn't want to stretch out all the way. This made for some challenges in this position, but I was able to strike a compromise by pointing my left knee out and slightly bending the leg. I found that I couldn't stay in this position for too long, but it did provide a nice respite from the other two positions. I may have even fallen asleep in this position one or two times.

My preferred sleeping position both before the accident and afterwards is pointing to the right. In my case, the left knee was slightly elevated in this position and this eliminated any weight being placed on it. Somewhat interestingly, the most comfortable position that I was able to discover was one in which I was positioned close to the edge of the bed and I would drape my left knee down and over the edge of the bed. In this position, the left knee was dangling in space and was not resting on anything. I found that this provided me with the best chance to forget about my knee for a while.

As a middle-aged man, I can tell you that I am not able to make it through a night without having to get up and use the bathroom at some point in time. It turns out that this is quite the challenge: the room is dark, you are sleepy, and you need assistance to move around.

I kept my crutches close to the bed for just such occasions. When nature called, I would get up grab my crutches and then take very slow, small, careful steps as I headed to the bathroom. I did not want to fall or bump into anything. One of the bigger challenges of this journey was coming out of the bathroom when I would click the light off. I'd be plunged into darkness and would not be able to see anything for a while. I'd find myself standing in the middle of the bathroom waiting for my eyes to adjust to the darkness. I had to be careful to not fall asleep standing up or I could have fallen over.

Oh, and one more thing — leg tremors. This is the strangest thing. I'm not exactly sure why these occur; however, I suspect that it has something to do with the fact that you are not using your leg. However, as you lay in your bed, every so often you'll have a bout of "leg tremors". During one of these tremors, the muscles in your leg are going to alternately tighten up and then release. A tremor does not generally last that long, but it can be quite unnerving and you'll be disturbed to discover that you really have no control over it — you'll just have to ride it out.

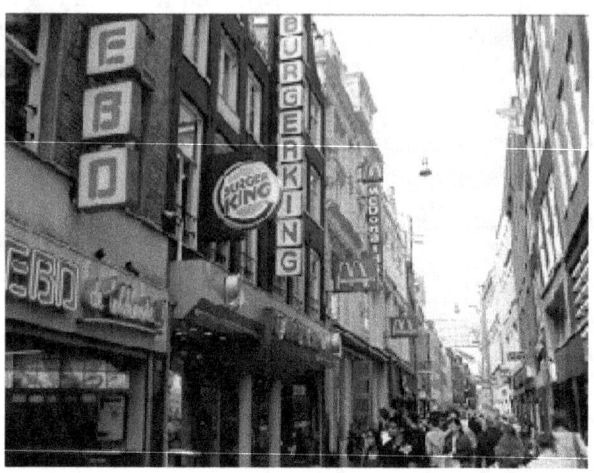

4.8 Eating Out

So when you have a broken leg, there are a lot of things that you cannot do. However, eating out is not one of them. Now, I must confess in the early days of my recovery the last thing in the world that I really wanted to do was to go to the effort of going out to eat. However, I quickly realized that this was a key part of the normal flow of life for my family. If I was going to have any hope of helping them to get over my traumatic injury and get back to their normal lives, then I needed to make the effort to restore this part of the family routine.

So let's look at what is involved in going out to eat if you are on crutches. First, there will be getting into whatever vehicle that you'll be going in. Depending on how much time you've been spending in a car, this may not be such a big deal. In my case it meant making it out of the house and into the family minivan.

My wife would be driving and I would be responsible for loading myself into the passenger seat. Note that being driven around all the time is just a bit emasculating. Additionally, when I reached the van, I had to deal with the challenge of where to put my crutches. I opted for opening the door behind the front seat and just shoving them in there on the floor. The thinking was that this way they were readily available when I got out.

When we got to the restaurant, my wife would often pull up to the door and then wait for me to get out. I would then reverse the process that I had gone through to get into the van — retrieve the crutches and then go hobbling off. What I discovered is that some restaurants have a ramp for handicapped people to gain access to the front door and some don't.

Of even more interest from my point-of-view was if they had modified their sidewalk to permit easy access from the parking lot — creating a ramp up the sidewalk. If this was available, I would take it. The alternative was for me to approach the sidewalk, stand on my good foot, and very much like getting in the shower I would place both crutch ends up on the sidewalk, and move the broken foot over the sidewalk and then "pop" up with the good leg. It worked, but it was not pretty.

Once inside the restaurant, everything proceeded normally. However, the one additional challenge that I had was to find a place to put my crutches. I had to make sure that the server would not be tripping over them and that I could easily get to them. Laying them up against the table worked well most times. However, an even better solution was when I could somehow place them under the table. They were out of the way for everyone and I didn't have to worry about them falling.

One interesting take-away that I have from my "eating out while on crutches" adventure is that I still have a negative impression of the first place that we went out to eat at. I can't actually tell you if the food was poor or it was just my attitude with life. The effort, the constant danger of falling, the feeling of being a burden on everyone who was with me, etc. all contributed to a sour attitude on my part. This was despite the fact that I should have been happy to just be getting out of the house! No matter, I've not been back to that restaurant since that visit and I can't really blame them. Be careful where you go!

Although crutches are quite handy, there are still a number of challenges that you'll face when using them. Somewhat interestingly, the most dangerous surface that I encountered during my three months of using crutches was in the restroom of a restaurant called "Twin Peaks" which is located in Orlando, Florida.

The floor was made of some sort of rubbery material that probably makes it very easy to clean a restroom floor, but when you are on crutches this floor surface came across as very slippery and I had a great deal of difficulty getting any grip on it with my rubber tips. Whenever I found myself in a situation where I was concerned about my safety while on my crutches, my "walking" technique changed. I started taking much smaller "steps" and I worked very hard to keep my crutches as straight up and down as possible. This allowed me to put almost my full body weight on the crutches in an effort to drive them into the ground as much as possible and prevent any slipping out the sides. Keep your eyes open when you're out!

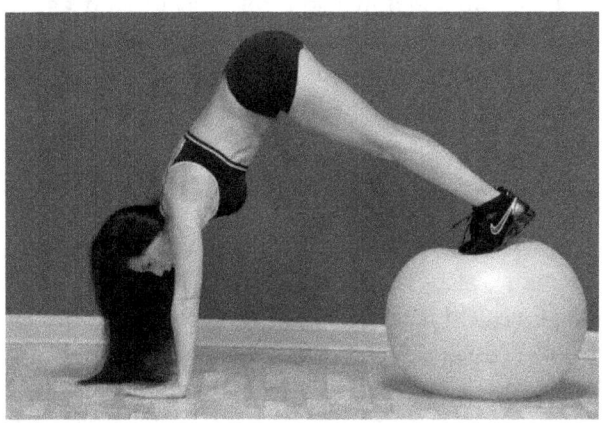

5   Exercising

I suspect that you are not going to want to hear this, but when you break a leg, you have suddenly signed yourself up for a new job: exercise. As you will very quickly become aware of, no matter how active or inactive you used to be before the accident, when you break a leg you will suddenly become a lot less active by necessity. If you don't take immediate action, then you are going to discover the true meaning of the word "atrophy". What this means is that the leg that you have broken is suddenly no longer being used. This will cause the muscles, tendons, and ligaments in that leg to start to shrink up and in some cases waste away. There is nothing that you can do to completely stop this from happening; however, you can take steps to minimize it.

If you need motivation to take the time to exercise, then allow me to give it to you. Once you are permitted to once again put your weight on your broken leg, you will instantly start to stretch the muscles, tendons, and ligaments that have remained dormant (for three months in my case). How can I clearly communicate the sense of pain that you will experience when you do this? It not only hurts, but it hurts a lot. Just imagine every single step that you take causing shooting pains to run both up and down your formally broken leg. There you go — that's what you are looking at. I don't think that there is anything that you can do to prevent this from happening; however, the more that you exercise, the better prepared your broken leg will be to resume it's normal activities and your time of pain will be not eliminated, but at least minimized.

One of the questions that will come up quickly will be "how long is all of this going to take?" What you are really asking is how long it is going to take until you once again walk normally. I've got two depressing stats for you: 44% of the people who have broken a leg reported that one year after the break they were still not walking normally. Additionally, my doctor told me multiple times that I should expect my recovery to take up to a year.

Now, I'm an engineer and I didn't like knowing that I was going to be broken for that long. I worked long and hard at my recovery. Not crazy like, but hard: after I was permitted to once again walk on my formally broken leg I would take stairs every chance I got and I went for three half-mile walks every day after each meal. Every day. It's my belief that a non-crazy dedicated person can expect to spend a month recovering for every month that they spent on crutches. In my case this meant three months of dedicated recovery efforts.

Your recovery will not be linear. What I mean by this is that when I first started to walk, it was uncomfortable. However, over time I got better and it hurt less. However, roughly a month and a half into my walking program something wonderful / horrible happened. A whole bunch of major muscles that apparently had not been previously involved in the walking program decided to get involved. My walking overnight became slow and painful once again. I say that this was wonderful because I believe that every time that you take a step and it hurts, you are stretching something that needs to be stretched and if you do it often enough then it will stop hurting and start helping your walking. Sorta a mixed blessing. I was sad that my walking had deteriorated so far, but I kept at it. I had a very bad week with a lot of pain and discomfort but I walked through it. At the end of the week, the pain went away and I was once again walking better than I ever had. You'll probably have to go through something like this, but take it from me — you are making progress and you need to keep at it!

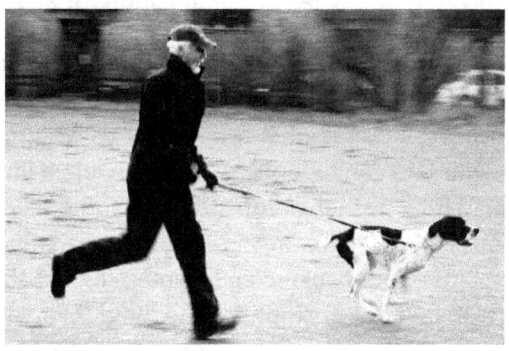

5.1   Why Exercise?

I'm lazy. I suspect that given a choice (especially after breaking a leg) you'd like to be lazy also. Alas, that is not in the cards for us because we have a lot of exercise ahead of us. However, before starting this undertaking, maybe we should have a quick discussion about just exactly why you are going to be putting the time in to exercise. I mean, exercise is not fun under the best of circumstances and this is most defiantly not the best of circumstances. Let's make sure that you understand why you'll be doing this.

Somewhat interestingly, one of the main reasons for embarking on a program of exercise is because you don't want to look bad in front of your doctor. After surgery (or whatever treatment you had), you can expect to be meeting with your orthopedic surgeon roughly every 30 days or so. At each of these meetings he / she will be looking at X-rays of your leg in order to ensure that the bones are healing correctly and they will also be looking at the leg in general. When they do this, they'll be interested in how well the leg bends. Trust me on this one — if you are not exercising, then that leg is NOT going to be bending. They will first want you to get to be able to do a 90 degree bend, and then they'll want more from you. I believe that I eventually got up to what I would call a 135 degree bend and I was quite proud of myself. However, at the 135 mark it really hurt to hold my leg in that position for any length of time!

Sleeping is the next reason that you are going to want to engage yourself in a program of exercise. At night you'll stretch yourself out in your bed and that's when you'll discover just how far you can extend your broken leg. If you have not been exercising it, then if you stretch it too far, it will start to hurt. You really don't want to be woken up in the middle of the night because your broken leg is screaming out that you've left it in a stretched out position for too long! If you do exercise, then you'll have a wider range of possible sleeping positions that you'll be able to sink into and remain asleep when you do.

Finally, you have a goal. You may not have realized that you have a goal, but you do. You want to be able to walk normally again as soon as possible. At the three month point in my recovery my doctor answered my question about how long it would take for me to walk normally again by telling me that it could take up to a full year. A full year? No way! This provided me with the motivation to do my exercises so that when I could walk again I could more quickly start to work on walking normally again.

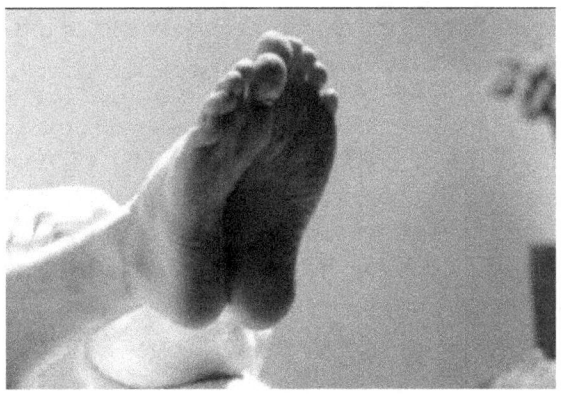

5.2   Types Of Exercises That You Can Do

So you've got a broken leg. Just exactly what kind of exercises are your medical caregivers expecting you to perform? I mean, your leg is broken so jogging, lifting weights, and that darn treadmill are all out. This is, of course, the place that I remind you that you need to talk with your medical team before starting any program of exercise that I may discuss with you. They know your specific situation and your circumstances and so they are in the best position to make the recommendations that will work the best for you.

However, with all of that being said, what we're talking about is a series of non-weight bearing exercises that are designed to keep the stretchy things in your leg from wasting away and to allow you to start to rebuild some of the muscle that you have undoubtedly lost by now.

The first one of these exercises is a foot flex. This is a simple exercise that you can do sitting in a chair with your broken leg up on a footstool or another chair and out in front of you. Simply take your foot and attempt to point forward as far as you possibly can with your big toe. Your foot will rock forward on your heel and you'll feel not only the muscles in your foot start to stretch but also the muscles in the front of your calf start to stretch also. When I would do this exercise, I would generally do it for 20 repetitions.

The next exercise that will be on your list is foot rotations. I discovered this exercise when I was doing a YouTube search of how people learned to walk again after breaking their leg. A guy had made a video of him doing the exercises that had been suggested to him by his physical therapist in the Netherlands.

In order to perform this exercise, you once again have to be sitting down in a chair. Your broken leg needs to be out in front of you on a footstool or another chair. Start by twisting your foot in a counterclockwise direction. Try to make the circle that you are making as big as possible. You'll want to do this 20 times. Once you are done with this, you now need to do exactly the opposite thing: you'll want to make 20 clockwise circles with your foot, once again making the circles as big as possible.

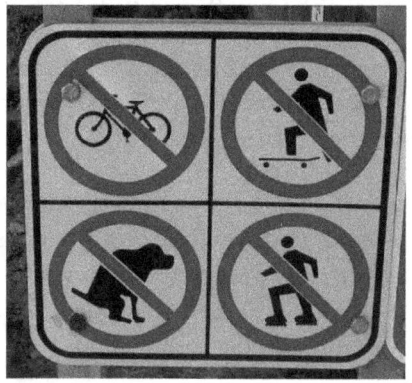

5.3   What You Can't Do

One of the most obvious things about exercising with a broken leg is that, at least initially, you are not going to be able to put any weight on the broken leg. It turns out that this is actually a very big deal. During the time that you are "off" of your broken leg (in my case this was 90 days), a number of very interesting things are going to happen to the leg — most of them not good. Yes, with a little luck your broken bones will start to stitch themselves back together. However, at the same time two very bad things will be happening. The first will be the onset of osteoporosis and the second will be what happens to all of the stretchy things in your leg.

The onset of osteoporosis in the broken leg is actually to be expected if you understand how the body works. Under normal circumstances the daily pounding that your bones take is a good thing. The constant compression that each bone gets put through several times a day causes the bone to react by creating more bone material. This means that just by walking or jogging, you are making your skeleton stronger.

While your broken leg heals and you are not walking on it, the bones in that leg will not be getting the normal shocks that they are used to. The bones won't be getting any stronger and in fact they will start to weaken through disuse. The only good news that I have for you here is that this process will be relatively quickly reversed once you start to walk again. Just make sure that you protect the formally broken leg for a while because it will be weaker than all of the other bones in your body.

The other not so nice thing that will be going on while you hobble around on crutches is that all of the stretchy parts of your leg (muscles, tendons, and ligaments) will not be used for the time that you are on the crutches. In an amazingly short amount of time they will then start to shrink up on you. You probably won't recognize that this is happening unless you start to see that bending your leg is becoming harder and harder to do. You will become very, very aware of all of the shrinkage that has occurred once you start to walk. You'll struggle to stretch out your leg, it won't be strong enough to hold you, and various muscle groups will trigger every time you take a step.

What all of this means for you is that the exercises that you can do while you are waiting for permission to once again put weight on your broken leg are that much more important. You need to do everything in your power to make sure that your broken leg retains as much of its flexibility as you can. Trust me on this, the alternative is quite painful.

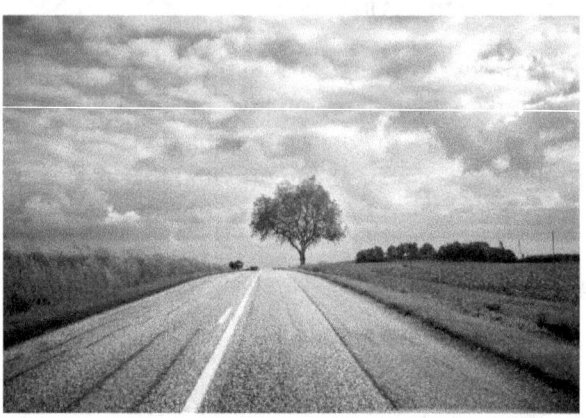

6   The Road To Recovery

The goal of anyone who has broken a leg is to recover as quickly as possible. However, what we all discover is that even though the accident may have happened very quickly, the recovery is something that is going to take a long time. We are going to go through a great deal of change during this time and if we don't know what to expect there is a good chance that it's going to leave us angry and confused.

Why can't we do what we want to do when we want to do it? It turns out that there is a lot going on during our recovery and the more that we understand the process, the better we are going to be able to deal with and help it move along faster.

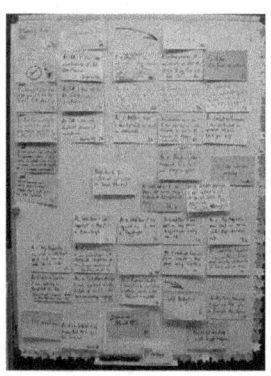

6.1 What Happens While You Heal: The 90-Day Plan

So after the injury and potentially after any surgery that you have to have, you now get down to the real task at hand: healing. The most important part of the healing process is to make sure that your bone(s) which have been broken are provided with an opportunity to heal correctly.

Shortly after your injury when you are in the care of a medical professional, they are going to be working to line your bones up correctly. Their goal is to fit the two part of the broken bone back together again so that they are touching. In some cases this is easy to do (no surgery) and some cases require some additional hardware to get things to stay in place (surgery).

No matter, once the bone pieces are touching, your body can get to work. Some of the bone around the area of the breakage has probably died by now. All the repair of your broken bone is going to be handled by your body's blood supply.

What most of us don't realize is that when we break a bone, we are also tearing the blood vessels associated with the bone that we broke. These blood vessels are the ones who carry nutrients to our bones. When you broke your bone, your body reacted immediately. There was swelling, blood pooled in the area, and you felt pain. The next step happens over the next few days. Your blood vessels will start to regrow in order to reconnect with each other. At the same time, the area where the break happened will be filled by a soft callus that the body has created.

This soft callus is what rejoins the bones. After a few weeks (now you know why you are going to be on those crutches for 90 days!) the soft callus will become a hard callus. The final stage in this process occurs over the next few months as the hard callus (or "bony callus") gets remodeled by the body to become fine bone. After this stage has been completed, it will actually be quite difficult to even tell where the fracture occurred.

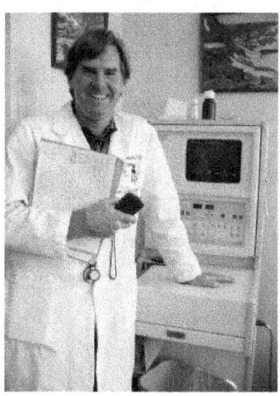

6.2   Visits To the Doctor

An important part of any recovery will be your visits to the doctor. You should expect to have at least three visits to the doctor over the roughly three months that it is going to take your bones to heal. Each one of these visits will be similar to the others and with a little luck the doctor will not have too much to tell you. What they are going to be looking for are any issues that you have run into. This is truly a case where you want your doctor to be bored when he or she meets with you!

Clearly the first visit after surgery, if that's what you needed, will be the most important. The last time this doctor saw you he/she had you opened up and they were manipulating your bones. Their interest now is going to primarily be in how your wound is healing. In my case, I had two wounds that needed to heal. The primary one was a seven inch scar in the form of a reversed number 7 which is where he had put a 5" piece of metal in and screwed it to the two parts of my bone that had separated.

During the operation a guide wire (perhaps for the holes in the bone that had been pre-drilled for screws to be inserted?) had gotten away from him. To retrieve it, he had had to make another much smaller opening on the back of the knee that he was working on.

The large wound, the 7" one, had been stapled shut after the operation was over. What this meant for me is that those staples had to be removed. At the third meeting with the doctor, his medical assistant said that she'd be removing the staples.

What this meant is that she would apply a numbing agent, wait a moment, and then pull one set of staples out of my leg. This went pretty well, but the numbing agent didn't work as well the further that she got into this process and so I defiantly felt the last few staples being removed!

After the staples were removed, small gauze bandages were placed over the wound in order to keep it shut. These turned out to be amazing bandages because despite taking a shower every day, they just would not fall off like they were supposed to. After way too much time had elapsed, my wife finally became fed up with them and removed them.

In my recovery, I got lucky and despite the fact that wounds on the lower part of your leg are high risk wounds because your blood flow to this area is limited, I ran into no problems.

Your visits to the doctor should be treated as the special events as they are. Despite reading this book and gaining the knowledge that I am sharing with you, you'll still have a bunch of questions about your specific recovery. You are going to want to write these questions down as they pop into your head so that you can remember to ask them to your doctor.

I had a lot of them. A number of my questions revolved around why the knee on my broken leg appeared to be so much larger (and puffy) than my other knee. I also asked a lot of questions about my final state: would I be able to jog, would I walk with a limp, could I expect to recover fully? These were questions that I suspect that he got from all of his patients and so he did a great job of providing me with the information that I was looking for.

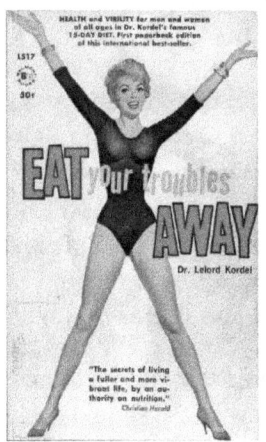

6.3　Diet

Darn that leg. Now what is there to eat? You've suffered a serious injury and what you choose to eat after your injury / surgery is going to play an important role in helping you to get better quicker.

When I injured myself one of the first things that I did was to hop onto the Internet and start to do some research on what I should be eating in order to minimize my recovery time. I, of course, found what I was looking for right off the bat. It turns out that your body is going to be working very hard in order to repair your broken bone. What this means is that you are now responsible to make sure that you provide your body with the calories that it will need to fuel this repair effort.

What I found on the Internet told me that I now needed to adopt a "high calorie diet". Tell me no more! If you were on a diet before your accident, officially consider yourself now off of it. During your recovery time, the first 90 days at least, you need to fuel the repair machine and so making sure that you are eating enough will be critical.

I do have a confession to make here. Upon discovering that I needed to adopt a high calorie diet, I started going to my local Dairy Queen restaurant and getting a delicious ice-cream snack every day. Eventually my wife started helping me out.

It turns out that Dairy Queen makes 14 different flavors of Blizzard treats. I started cycling through this list during my 90 days immediately following my surgery. I know that you want to know what impact this had on my body. I'm here to tell you that my high-calorie diet combined with my inability to engage in any real physical exercise resulted in me gaining roughly 15 pounds during the 90 days that I was on crutches.

One of the most fascinating things that I discovered when I was researching what I should eating was that my broken bones were going to rebuild themselves no matter what I ate. However, how they did it was going to depend very much on what I ate. One of the fundamental building blocks of a bone is, of course, calcium. If your body can't get enough of this stuff in order to repair your broken bones then it's going to have to go find it elsewhere.

Calcium and amino acids are mobilized from other body stores in response to skeletal injury. What this means for you is that your body will start to leach calcium from your other bones and then use it to repair your broken bone. Yes, you'll heal the broken bone; however, at the same time you are going to end up weakening your other bones.

Your rate of bone loss can double while your body is repairing your broken bone. I think that we can all agree that this is not something that any of us wants to have happen. In order to prevent this from happening, you are going to have to ensure that your diet while you are on the mend contains what your body is going to need in order to fix itself.

What you need to understand is that the rebuilding of a broken bone will go through four different and distinct phases.

The first is called Inflammation and it's where your body releases blood that is used to build an initial spongy bridge between the two pieces of broken bone. The next phase is called Repair and this is when the spongy bridge is turned into a hard callous that joins the two pieces of bone together in a rough fashion with bumps and such.

The next phase is called Remodeling and this is where the body reshapes the rough join of the two bone pieces and makes them look more like the bone used to look. The final phase is called Maintenance and this is where the body simply manages the repaired bone.

So just exactly what should your diet now start to include? The first component will be vitamin D. Vitamin D is a fat-soluble vitamin that is naturally present in very few foods, added to others, and available as a dietary supplement. It is also produced endogenously when ultraviolet rays from sunlight strike the skin and trigger vitamin D synthesis.

Vitamin D promotes calcium absorption in the gut. It is also needed for the later stages of healing, the Remodeling and the Maintenance phases, where it promotes bone growth and bone remodeling. Without sufficient vitamin D, bones can become thin, brittle, or misshapen. The recommended amount of vitamin D that we should be getting is between 600 and 1,500 International Units per day. However, the average adult between ages 20-60 generally gets less than 200 International Units per day.

Calcium is another important part of any diet following a bone break. Calcium, the most abundant mineral in the body, is found in some foods, added to others, available as a dietary supplement, and present in some medicines (such as antacids). 99% of the body's calcium supply is stored in the bones and teeth where it supports their structure and function.

Bone itself undergoes continuous remodeling, with constant resorption and deposition of calcium into new bone. It is recommended that we get 1,200 mg of calcium each day in either our diet or supplements. Unfortunately, studies have shown that the median dietary intake of calcium by women over 40 is about 600 mg and for men it is about 900 mg.

Vitamin C has been shown to improve fracture healing in animal and human studies. Vitamin C helps your body produce collagen which forms connective tissue and is used to heal the broken bone. Vitamin C will be most helpful during the Repair phase of the healing process. Studies have shown that we benefit from extra levels of vitamin C during the fracture healing process.

It is recommended that we get 85 mg per day of vitamin C. However, the median intake of vitamin C for adults between the ages of 20-60 is 60 mg per day.

Vitamin E is another needed component of your healing diet. Vitamin E is found naturally in some foods, added to others, and available as a dietary supplement. "Vitamin E" is the collective name for a group of fat-soluble compounds with distinctive antioxidant activities. Vitamin E is involved in immune function and, as shown primarily by in vitro studies of cells, cell signaling, regulation of gene expression, and other metabolic processes.

Additional items that you may want to add to your diet (that I added to mine) include L-Arginine and L-Lysine. L-arginine is a nonessential amino acid increases blood flow through the coronary artery. L-arginine is a chemical building block called "an amino acid." It is obtained from the diet and is necessary for the body to make proteins. L-arginine is found in red meat, poultry, fish, and dairy products. It can also be made in a laboratory and used as medicine. L-arginine is used for heart and blood vessel conditions.

Finally, a general multi-vitamin may also be added to your diet. The studies have shown that most of us really don't need an everyday multivitamin; however, during your healing process you need to make sure that your body is being provided with all of the building blocks that it is going to be needing.

Remember, on top of the normal process of keeping your body running smoothly, you are now asking your body to take on the additional task of repairing a broken bone. You'd like to have this task completed without compromising any of the other systems in your body. Stating things off by eating the correct diet is a good way to make sure that you end up with the results that you are looking for.

6.4   Do More As Soon As You Can

You won't be on crutches forever and as the end of the three month period (or whatever your time frame is) approaches, you'll start to get antsy to start walking again. I can tell you that my orthopedic surgeon scared me so badly about what would happen if I tried to walk too soon that I really was not tempted to try walking until he gave the ok.

However, I did develop what I called my "fake walking" technique. What this consisted of was my placing my broken left foot fully on the floor and making it "look" like I was walking on it. In reality all of the weight was supported by my wrists. However, it did give my broken leg an opportunity to once again go through the motions of walking without violating the doctor's orders. Doing this probably also helped to prevent me from trying to walk on my own before being giving permission to do so by my doctor.

In my case, when my doctor finally gave me the green light to start to put weight on my broken leg once again, you can well imagine how overjoyed I was! It was his suggestion that I stay on the crutches for a while, then I could transition to one crutch and when I felt ready, I could switch to using a cane. I thanked the doctor for his input, went home and promptly threw my crutches away.

I got out my cane and went for a lurching walk around my neighborhood (perhaps about 1/2 of a mile). I'd say that I used the crutch for about two weeks until one day I realized that I no longer needed it. I will confess that I kept the cane handy. In certain circumstances I would use it — it's amazing how helpful people will be when they see you approaching and using a cane!

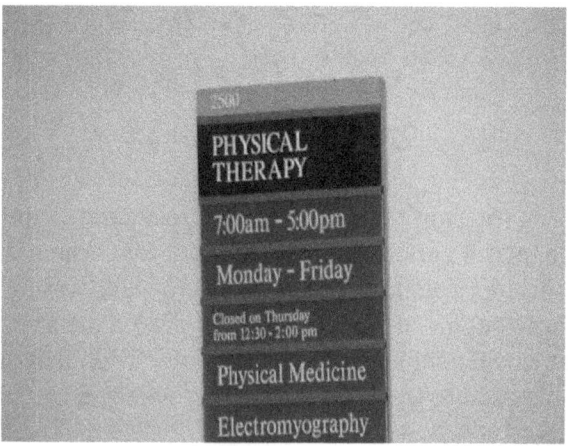

6.5 Physical Therapy

While you are on crutches, there is not much that can be done to help you walk better. However, once your doctor gives you the green light and tells you that you can start to put weight on the broken leg again, this is when the real work begins. In my case, during the meeting with my doctor where he said that I could start to walk again, I asked him if I needed to sign up for some physical therapy. His answer surprised me. He told me that in my case physical therapy was not needed.

He said that he would be prescribing it if I was either obese or elderly. He said that the primary reason to send people to physical therapy after breaking a limb is because the doctor does not believe that they will start to use the limb again. It's going to hurt to walk again, at least initially. My doctor's thinking was that he knew that I was eager to start walking again and so I didn't need a physical therapist pushing me to walk — I'd do it on my own.

That being said, once I started walking again, it turned out that I had a lot to learn. The very first thing that I had to master was how to walk. You might think that this is just something that we all already know how to do. However, when you have not been using a leg to walk for three months it can be amazing what you forget how to do. In my case, I discovered that instead of walking correctly, I was doing an odd sort of shuffle step. In order to get things right, I had to sit down and think about what the correct way to walk is.

It turns out that there are four parts to a correct step. First your heel comes into contact with the ground. Next the pad of your foot (the part just before your toes) comes into contact with the ground. Finally, your toes come into contact with the ground. The final part of a step is when your toes push off of the ground. In order to walk correctly, I discovered that I had to think through all four phases each time my formally broken leg was used to walk. Over time this did not take as much concentration; however, I did discover myself slipping back into the shuffle step sometimes and once again I had to focus on the right way to walk.

How much are you going to have to walk before you can walk normally? That's a really good question. I believe that you are not going to be approaching a normal gait until you have taken the time reacquaint your leg with how to walk. Clearly this is not going to happen in a day, a week, or even a month. The good news is that every time you take a step you will be getting just a bit better. I believe that you need to take 10,000 steps (roughly 3 months of walking) before you'll have a relatively normal looking walk.

I believe that how you start out walking once you are given permission to do so is very important — this is going set the stage for your full recovery. You have been dreaming about walking ever since you broke the leg and once you can do it you are going to want to run out there and get to it. However, you'll quickly discover that this simply is not possible. Your leg has been both damaged and not been used for a period of time and because of that it no longer works the way that it used to.

In my case what this meant was that I was not able to walk unaided. Instead of having to use crutches, I was now able to get by using a cane. Sort of. Initially walking with a cane was very painful and slow work. Every time I put weight on my leg I had shooting pains go up my leg. Since I had spent three months with my leg off the ground and slightly bent at all times, I was no longer able to easily fully extend it. This meant that I had a very pronounced limp as I walked. Yes, I could walk with a cane, but no, it was not a pretty sight.

I realized that I was at the start of a long journey that I wanted to attempt to complete as quickly as possible. In my case I knew that I could walk around the block where I live and each time I would be covering roughly 1/2 of a mile. There were some social issues here: my neighbors saw me walking and the all offered their condolences.

The up side to this was that as the days and weeks went by, I got better at walking with my cane. My neighbors noticed and I received many complements on how fast I was improving. Having a fixed walking path and knowing that I would traversing it twice a day allowed me to feel that I was making progress in my recovery every day.

One of the things that may not be initially obvious to the recovering broken leg individual is that one of their greatest challenges is going to come in the form of stairs. When you are climbing or descending stairs, you are placing your entire body weight on the formally broken leg. This can hurt a great deal.

Every single step either up or down a staircase will be very uncomfortable. However, with this being said, taking the stairs when you have this option is a great idea. Yes, I understand that you won't want to because of the discomfort involved, but you need to realize that you have to work through the discomfort to get to where you want to be. Taking the stairs when you have a chance is a great way to give your broken leg an intense workout each time you do it.

Once you start walking you may think that you no longer have to do your stretching exercises. That would be incorrect. The stretching exercises will continue to allow you to push your leg muscles further than just walking will. Your goal here is to get all of the various parts of your leg system to stretch out just like they were before the accident.

Walking is going to help this happen, but walking is simply going to be you using the muscles that you have already used. Stretching is going to extend the envelope that you can move your leg in and as this increases, you'll automatically start to use the new mobility both when you are walking and when you are climbing stairs.

As important as it is to try to walk as much as you can, you need to realize that when you are not walking your formally broken leg will tend to start to tighten up on you once again.

This will be most evident when you first get up in the morning and experience the worst walking of the day.

Additionally, if you happen to go on a long car ride when you first get out of the car you will probably be limping for the first few steps that you take. Realize that this will happen and, if you can, attempt to stretch out your leg before trying to walk on it. You will probably still experience some discomfort and limping, but it will go away quickly the more stretching that you can do.

As you work to get your leg back into shape, there is an important point that you need to realize. Simply put, your leg is very complex system. This means that it is made up of a number of different subsystems that each consist of different groups of muscles, tendons, and ligaments. You'll discover this as you start to walk again. On any given day, you may discover that there is a new part of your leg that is causing you discomfort.

What will happen (hopefully) is that you'll keep walking even though there is a great deal of discomfort. Over time, the parts of the leg that are hurting will hurt less. Unfortunately, what will now happen is that a new group of muscles will then start to speak up and let you know that they are now starting to participate in the walking process and they will start to hurt you. This process will go on for a good three months as you continue to walk more and more.

All of this naturally leads to a question that I suspect you've never really spent a great deal of time thinking about. Just exactly how should you be walking? I mean, before the accident you would just get up and walk. Now that you are in your recover phase, you really can't walk like you used to so how should you be trying to walk. What should your goal be?

I'm hoping that you've watched as much television as I have over the years. The reason that this is now so important is because I'm going to tell you that I think that you should be striving to walk like an English gentleman. Hmm, just exactly what does that mean?

In a word, good posture. This means that your back should be straight up and down, your shoulders should be squared, and your head should be held high and you should be looking forward. As simple as all of this sounds, it's actually fairly hard to do when you are limping along on a leg that used to be broken. However, if you can keep a mental image of what an English gentleman looks like when he is walking in your head, then you'll know what you should be shooting for.

The process of walking will now consist of you rolling your foot when you walk: curl the toes and push off at the end of each step. This is not easy to do and will require some mental concentration to remember to do it with each step. The good news is that the more that you walk, you'll start to see improvements.

One of the first improvements that you are going to be seeing is that your walking speed is going to start to speed up. Your first few walks are going to be painful and slow. However, over time the discomfort will start to settle down and your pace will pick up. Do be careful when you are using stairs at this stage of the game. You are going to want to keep a careful eye on where your feet are being placed. A misstep now can become very painful.

In my case, over time my walking with a cane improved. Eventually I was still taking the cane with me, but not using it. I would turn the cane upside down and tuck it behind my arm and just carry it. It was there if I become tired, but it was just slowing me down otherwise. One final note was that during this phase of your recovery you may be dealing with constant pain. You've probably used up any painkillers that were given to you by your doctor or the hospital. The good news is that I found that taking one Alieve in the morning will help you to deal with walking pain

In this book I generally try to focus both on the things that you can do and just exactly how you can go about doing them. However, in order to be realistic, we need to realize that there will be some things that you are just not going to be able to do during your recovery period. The good news is that as you heal, these things will once again become something that you can do. However, you have to realize that you do have limitations and you need to be careful to not and try to overdo it.

One of the most basic things that you will quickly discover that is now beyond your ability to do is the simple task of picking things up. When you are on crutches, both of your hands are going to be fully occupied moving you around. You don't have any spare capacity to hold on to anything with your hands. You can do clever things like attach bags and such to your crutches, but this means that if you pick something up you'll need to place it into a bag before you start to move. Doing goofy things like trying to carry something in your hands and work your crutches with your armpits never works out so don't try it.

Walking dogs is also going to be something that is probably too much for you to handle right now. In my case, I have two 70 pound boxers and I did attempt to take them out into the yard while on crutches once. Let's just say that it did not end well — I ended up sitting on the front lawn holding onto a dog's leash as he strained to go somewhere else. Not a good story. If you have large animals, let someone else take care of them.

Finally, fixing things around the house is probably also out for now. Most home repair tasks require you to do a number of different tasks such as stand on ladders, reach up high, etc. Your crutches make you much wider right now and so there is a good chance that you are not going to be able to fit into small spaces. The fact that your leg probably does not bend right now also means that if you have to get down on the floor to perform a task, you're going to be dragging your leg behind you. All in all, your days as a handyperson have probably come to a halt during your initial recover period.

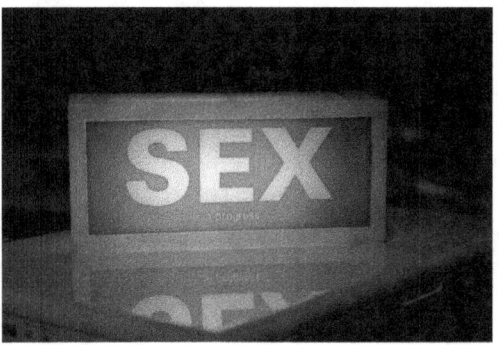

6.7   Sex

Ouch! Do we even need to talk about this? Well, yes. What's interesting here is that I really shouldn't be talking with you — I should be talking with your partner. For you see, you have suffered a traumatic injury. From the initial trip to the hospital, the wrapping of the damaged limb, potentially the surgery, the use of crutches and all of the things that you can no longer do while you are healing, your partner is probably looking at you differently these days. This is where the problems tend to start.

Your total recovery time from a broken limb can take up to a year. If you've had an active sex life before breaking your limb, that's a bit too long to take a break for. The problem here more often than not is that your partner now views you as being "made of eggshells". What this means is that they are afraid that if they get too close to you, they will end up hurting you in some way. This means that it's going to be up to you to clearly communicate to them what you are going to be capable of doing.

I don't really care just how randy you are. You are going to have to start things off slowly. You need to understand where they are coming from and you have to go meet them there. Start off simply by sitting together. Show them that your upper body is still quite mobile and does not cause you any problems.

If you are still on crutches, invite them to the bedroom, but ask that they follow you in a few minutes. This will allow you to hobble off to the bedroom, take care of things, set your crutches off to the side, and get into bed before they arrive. Preventing them from seeing you moving around on crutches can go a long way in convincing them that you are getting closer to being more like the person that you used to be.

Just exactly what happens during your intimate time with your partner is up to you. I would suggest that before anything starts that you take the time to think out the scenario that you would like to unfold. Understand that you probably are not going to be able to bend your leg. Kneeling on your knees is also probably out of the picture for right now. The good news is that you may be able to stand on one leg, lay on your chest, and, of course, lay on your back. Given what you can do, how do you want the evening to go?

After the interaction is over, you have a responsibility to communicate to your partner how things were for you. Clearly you are going to want to thank them for a good time. If there was some position or activity that caused you discomfort, this is the time to bring it up. Explain that you had not anticipated having a problem, but that you did. Ask for their input on what could be done differently the next time in order to prevent the same problem from showing up. By getting their input this way, you are setting the stage for your next romp between the sheets!

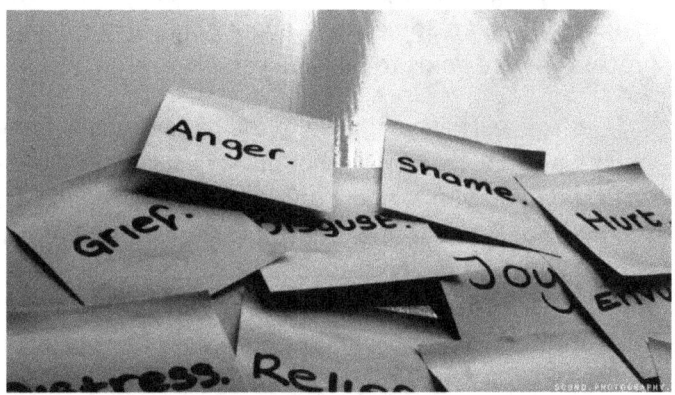

6.8　Emotional Issues

You wouldn't think that emotional issues would have any place in a book about how to heal a broken leg, but it does. It turns out that because it takes so long for a broken leg to heal, that both you and the people who are in your life will undergo a wide range of emotions that you need to both realize and deal with as they show up. You need to realize that quite naturally you are going to be feeling a great deal of anger that this broken leg has happened to you.

Like me, you'll probably run what happened through you head over and over again trying to determine what could have been done differently that would not have resulted in you breaking your leg. In my case I fell off of my bike in the middle of a rain storm. There was nobody else to blame and it was just fate that it happened. This did not stop me from going back the event in my mind and trying to come up with ways that I could have done things differently that would have prevented me from breaking my leg.

Over time this will fade and you'll accept what has happened to you. However, three months to heal a broken limb is a very long time for someone who used to be very active. Once the surgery, if required, is over and done with, now you'll just be playing a waiting game as you wait for your bones to mend themselves. Somewhere about half way through this process you are going to become very frustrated.

You will have adjusted to the handicapped lifestyle that you are now living. A big part of this adjustment will be the realization that you are now officially a handicapped person. You may not like that title, but you will realize that at least for right now it does fit you and your situation. At this point in time you are going to have to start dealing with a rising level of frustration. You will be reminded on a daily basis of all of the things that you cannot do such as carry things, climb ladders, etc. The time between now and when you'll be permitted to walk again seems to very long and the unfairness of it all can overwhelm you.

This frustration is something that you are going to have to find a way to deal with. Instead of focusing on how much longer you have to go, instead you need to focus on how far you have already come. In my case, I printed out a single page that had a year calendar on it. I then proceeded to circle the 90 day mark after my surgery and every day I would cross off a day. It didn't get me to my goal any faster, but as the list of crossed off days started to grow and grow I could appreciate how far I had come. I also numbered each day: how long had it been since I started this journey and how many days did I have left to go to reach 90 days. This helped me to understand exactly where I was.

One other thing that you are going to have to take some time and think about will be the other people in your life. If you have a significant other, then you need to realize that your injury has had a profound impact on them also. First, this has served as a reminder that you are not invincible. Someday something could happen to you and that is a harsh wakeup call for someone who had been enjoying each day as it came.

Next, the fact that there are now many things that you cannot do means that there are a lot of things that you cannot do with your partner. You have dramatically changed their life just as much as you have changed your life. In my case, while I was on crutches I could not take my dogs out, I could not tend to our swimming pool, I could not fix things around the house, I could not get things down out of the attic, and I could not empty and put away the contents of the dishwasher. Each one of these is trivial by itself, but when taken together they created a big burden that my wife suddenly had to shoulder.

What this means for you is that not only do you have to deal with all of the issues associated with having a broken leg, but you also have to realize the impact that you are having on the other people in your life. You need to take steps to lessen the burden that your situation is placing on them. In my case, the first thing that I did was to remind myself to tell my wife "thanks" more often for all of the things that she was now doing because I could not.

As I became more capable on my crutches, I did try to take on more of the tasks that I had had to give up. Taking the dogs out while on crutches turned out to be a disaster and so I cannot recommend that! However, I found that I could empty the dishwasher and put the plates away. It was not easy, but with a bit of effort it could be done. This once again was trivial, but every little bit helps. Look for ways to show your appreciation and then take on tasks as your skills and mobility improve.

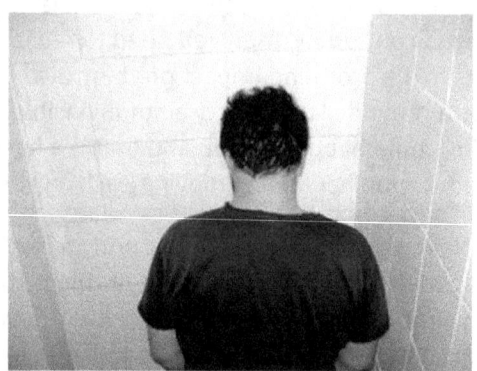

6.9   Urine

No, this is not a pleasant topic, but it is an important one that we should talk about: urine. If you end up having surgery, the issue of urine will start in the hospital. Now, I must confess that I can only address this topic from the standpoint of a male — I suspect that there may be some differences for females.

In the hospital after you've had your leg operated on, the one thing that they really don't want you to be doing is standing up and walking around. The primary reason that you would do this would be to go to the bathroom. To help you out with this, they'll provide you with a rather unique curved bottle that can hold let's say about 1/2 of a gallon. The thinking is that instead of getting up to go to the bathroom, you can just turn over on your side and very carefully (don't spill!) pee into the bottle.

The good news, if indeed there is any good news when we are talking about urine, is that the hospital is going to provide you with this urine bottle when you go home. The reason that this is such a big deal is because when you are at home, you are going to be facing the same problem that you faced in the hospital: a journey to the bathroom is a major effort.

In my life, the hospital bottle became my friend in two situations: when I was watching TV and when I was sleeping. I live in a crowded house so we're not going to talk about the TV situation too much, but needless to say that I had a blanket covering my lap and that's all that I have to say about that.

At night, I kept the container by my bed. In the first two months of being home from the hospital, it was my constant companion. When I woke up in the middle of the night and had to go, I would reach out and locate the container. I needed to be very careful because if I had already used it, it contained urine. I would then roll over to the side of the bed and while laying horizontal I would proceed to fill the container. Depending on how much liquid I had consumed before going to bed, the container could become quite full by morning.

Sometimes my partner would empty it out for me (talk about love!) and sometime that task would be left up to me. If I was going to empty it out, I would take the handle of the container and hook it onto the bar of one of my crutches and carry it into the bathroom that way in order to dump it out. An important thing to remember is that once it had been dumped out, it needed to be rinsed out and capped so that it didn't make the room smell like urine.

Over time I became convinced my laying down and filling my container was not the most efficient way to do things. I came to believe that this was resulting in me having to pee more times than I wanted to. I transitioned to sitting on the edge of the bed and filling my container. Over time I also came to believe that this was not the most efficient way to do things so that was when I started to crutch my way into the bathroom to go pee. Once I started walking again, I put the container away for good.

While we're talking about that bathroom, it's yet another place where there's a good chance that there will be some change in your life. I can tell you that prior to my accident, I was a fairly private person. I'd go into the bathroom, shut the door and do my business. However, once I started maneuvering around on crutches the simple act of going into the bathroom successfully became much more of a chore. Once I was there, I just wanted to do my business and leave.

It turns out that shutting the door when you are on crutches is a major effort: you have to twist around, reach out and grab some part of the door, and then attempt to yank it shut. When you are just paying a quick visit to the bathroom, this becomes way too much of an effort and you just start to leave the door wide open. You get my point here, when you have a broken leg, all manner of privacy in the bathroom gets thrown out the window.

Oh, one other thing. In my life my office is located on the 2nd floor of my house far away from any bathroom. If while I was working I decided that I needed to go to the bathroom, then I would have had to crutch over to the stairs, slide on down, crutch to the bathroom, and then repeat the process to get back to my desk. This would require a time investment of at least 5 minutes.

I decided to instead equip myself with a collection of 52 oz beverage cups from a local gas station and instead of making the trip downstairs I would simply stand up and partially fill one of these cups. It would take between 4-5 pees to fill a 52 oz cup. Now I had the problem that I could not carry these cups downstairs to flush them so I had talk my two boys into taking my "apple cider" downstairs so that I could get rid of it. Not pleasant, but it did solve the problem.

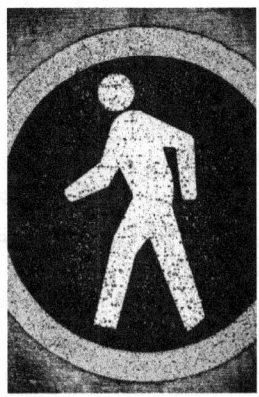

6.10 Walking Again

Ah the ultimate goal of anyone who has broken their leg: to walk once again. Hang, on it turns out that your body has been undergoing some significant changes while you've been laid up and you need to know about these. The ones that you'll be most cognizant of will be the muscle atrophy that has occurred in your broken leg. Just by looking at this leg you'll be able to see how much smaller it is than your other leg that has been moving you around for months.

One thing that has occurred that you won't be aware of is that you've experienced osteoporosis. The bones in the leg that you broke have become thinner and weaker. The way that bones grow is by the shock of you compressing and releasing them. While you've been on crutches this has not been happening and so the bones have suffered for it.

That magical day will finally arrive when your doctor tells you that you can now start to put weight on your formally broken leg! I had a discussion with my doctor about physical therapy and what he told me surprised me somewhat. He said that he was not going to recommend it for me (a middle aged man). He told me that in the case of a broken leg, physical therapy was generally only required for overweight or elderly patients. The thinking is that in these cases because it does hurt to walk, there is a very good chance that the patient won't make the effort to walk. The physical therapy is designed to force them to get up and walk,

He told me that he was confident that I would be getting up and walking without needing any extra motivation. The doctor told me that I'd probably want to switch from using two crutches to just using one. When I felt up to it, I could then switch to using a cane. I listened very carefully to what he told me and then I went home, threw away my crutches, got out my cane, and went for a walk around the neighborhood.

So what's walking going to be like? In short — it's not going to be pretty. Right off the bat you are going to look like a 90-year old man when you walk. It will hurt to put weight on your formally broken leg. You really won't want to do it. However, you will do it and then instantly regret that you just did it. I also discovered that there was a great deal of "lurching" to my walking, I was bent over and moving from side to side as I walked. I didn't want to walk like this forever and so I knew that I needed a walking role model.

I decided that I wanted to be able to walk like a proper English gentleman (as seen on TV and in the movies). This meant that I needed to walk with my spine straight, eyes forward, one leg in front of the other. This was not easy to do when my body was screaming for me to take smaller steps and to bend over in order to feel more comfortable. However, I was able to do it and slowly, very slowly, my walking started to look much more natural.

One of the thoughts that you'll have almost right off the bat is "how long is it going to take for me to start to walk the way I used to?" I'll remind you that my doctor told me that it can take up to 12 months to recover from a broken leg. This means that you're looking at potentially about 9 months to get walking back to normal. I've decided, and this is completely made up by me, that it takes 10,000 steps to get you back to walking normally.

What I've discovered is that every time that I go out for a walk, something else in my formally broken leg is uncomfortable. It may be a muscle in the foot itself, it may be part of the calf, etc. However, I have learned to be excited when I feel something new complaining in my leg. I know that this is some part of me that has not been stretched in a long time and once I exercise it, it will be one less thing that I'm going to have to worry about going forward.

This all brings up the interesting question that I suspect that most of us have not spent a lot of time thinking about: just exactly how do we go about walking. Let me tell you, this is going to be a question that you will now become very, very interested in getting an answer to. Walking has always been a part of our life and so we generally don't give it much thought. However, now that you are in the process of teaching yourself how to walk once again, you are going to have to relearn what you once knew by heart. Good news: I'm going to tell you how to walk. It turns out that taking a step, obviously, starts with you picking up your foot. Now, as it comes down, the first part of your foot that will make contact with the ground will be your heel. Generally, this is not a problem for you even now.

Next comes the pads that are on the bottom of your feet just before your toes. As you rock through your step, the next thing to come into contact will be your toes. This is where things start to feel uncomfortable for you. The final step (pardon the pun) in walking is for you to "spring" off of your toes as you launch your foot into the air once again to take a step. As you start to walk, you will feel a lot of different parts of your foot as you move thought these four parts of taking a step.

A key question that you might be asking is if you will still need to be doing any of the sitting down stretching exercises that you used to do before you were permitted to put weight on your formally broken leg. The answer is yes and no. I will confess that once I started walking, I stopped doing my sitting down stretching exercises. However, what I started to discover is that there were still positions that I could not stretch my leg into. Additionally, although I had been able to bend my leg back through about 135 degrees before I started walking, I felt as though I had lost some of this flexibility.

What I stated to do in order to help my walking was before getting up in the morning, I would go through three reps of two exercises. The first was to fully extend my formally broken leg and try to get it as straight as possible. This did not feel comfortable at all. Stretching it out caused a lot of things that had not been worked before to start to complain. After doing this for 30 seconds, I would then attempt to bend my leg as much as I could. 135 degrees was my goal and I was able to once again get there fairly quickly. At that amount of bending, the leg was not happy and would let me know about it. I would hold it in this position for roughly 30 seconds.

One of the biggest challenges with walking is trying to answer the question "am I making any progress?" Let me assure you that as you walk more and more, you will be making progress. Progress will come slowly and so it can be difficult to detect, but you'll notice it in a number of different areas. The first will be a reduction in the discomfort that you feel when you walk.

Initially, there will be a lot of complaining coming from your leg. Over time this will die down and only various muscles will be raising an objection. Next, your speed of walking will increase. When you first start to walk, you'll lurch down the sidewalk slowly as you anticipate the next bolt of pain that you'll get when you put the formally broken foot down again. As things improve, so will your rate of walking. No, you won't be going as fast as other people, but you will be going a lot faster than you did in the beginning.

Something that you may not realize right off the bat, but you soon will is that stairs are going to represent a unique challenge to you. The reason that stairs may be an issue in your life is because it turns out that you use a different set of leg muscles when you are both climbing and descending stairs. I suspect that you'll discover, just as I did, that climbing stairs is a uniquely painful experience.

There seem to be a set of muscles that are on top of the knee that are used to accomplish this task and just walking does not seem to exercise them. You are just going to have to work through this pain. Going down stairs causes a similar, but different experience. It's when you place your full body weight on your formally broken leg that you'll start to exercise muscles that have not been getting used. This will also be quite uncomfortable. I wish that I could tell you that I have some magic cure for these stair based muscle challenges; however, I don't. You just need to find as many stairs as you can and take the time to climb and descend them when you can.

All walking is not created the same. What I found is that the first few steps that you take are going to be the most painful and the most hesitant. When I stood up, I'd take just a moment and attempt to fully extend my formally broken leg. Then I'd take my first few steps. Those first steps are often painful and cause you to wobble just a bit. After you get moving, things will become better, but it will take time.

One of my biggest challenges came in the middle of the night. When I'd get up to use the bathroom, it was only a few steps away, but it was always those first few steps that I'd be taking in the dark when I was not fully awake. I found myself holding on to pieces of furniture and door frames for stability. Coming back to bed was always better because I had already taken my first few steps.

After I had been walking for a while, I started to study how I was walking more closely. What I discovered was that I had a nasty habit of walking slightly bent over, very much like you would expect an old man to walk. My question to myself was why I was doing this.

A little investigation revealed that I was not yet able to fully extend my broken leg — it was always at a roughly 5-10 degree angle. Because of this, when I put weight on the broken leg, I would tend to fall forward just a bit and this was causing me to bend over as I walked. With this realization, I knew what I had to do — I had to find a way to stretch the broken leg out so that it would be able to easily fully extend.

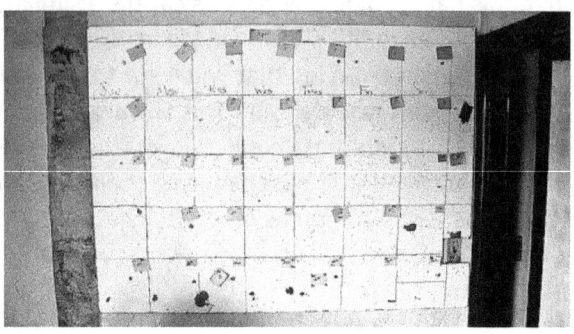

6.11 10 Months After The Accident

One of the big questions that I get asked is how aggressive was I in my recovery. I struggle with this question a bit because I really don't have anyone to measure myself against. However, in my head I picture one of those CrossFit people trying to recover from a broken leg and I can tell you that I was not that crazy. However, I think that I was probably just about a notch or two below them.

I started each day out in bed on my back stretching and bending my leg 90 times in order to limber it up. I would go for roughly 6 miles of walks every day once I was off of my crutches for a while. I would take two sets of stairs two or three times a day. I guess you could say that I was aggressive, but I was not crazy.

As an engineer, I had assumed that my walking would just keep getting better each and every day. It turns out that I was wrong. It turns out that I had my good days walking and my bad days. On good days, I could almost forget that I had broken my leg. Everything seemed to work together well and I felt no discomfort when I walked. On my bad days, I could feel every step.

I was constantly amazed that every day I was dealing with a new group of muscles that seemed to show up and call out for my attention. Sometimes it would be muscles located in the upper thigh, sometimes in the upper calf, and sometimes right over the knee. I never knew what tomorrow would bring. My thinking was that every time a new muscle showed up and started to complain about my walking, this was a good thing. As I walked more and more it would learn what it was supposed to be doing and it would eventually go away. This seemed to work, but there also seemed to be an unending stream of these muscles that just kept coming and coming.

One of my biggest challenges was stairs. I can't explain why, but for some reason the process of going up (and down) stairs caused me the most physical discomfort — and that's why I tried to do as much of it as possible. I suspect that the discomfort came from the fact that when you are taking the stairs, you bend the broken leg and then you transfer your whole body weight to it and then proceed to straighten it out. Doing this over and over again can cause some real discomfort. As I got better at taking the stairs, I started to take them two at a time in order to make my leg hurt even more. The thinking was that the more that it hurt, the quicker that it would heal.

During my recovery I would often take my two large dogs for a walk. What they taught me was that even though I was making progress in walking in a straight line, I still had a ways to go. Specifically, if I twisted or tried to move my leg while my foot was planted on the ground, I was going to be experiencing some real discomfort.

My dogs also taught me that I really could not run at this stage of my recovery. The best that I could do was to sort of do a peg leg hop that picked up my pace, but was still short of an actual run. I believe that a lot of my problems with moving faster came from the simple fact that I really could not easily bend the leg very much. This meant that any sort of speed increase resulted in me doing a sort-of peg-leg hopping action. This was not normally a critical issue, but when it started to rain and I was far away from any cover, I just had to realize that I was going to be getting wet.

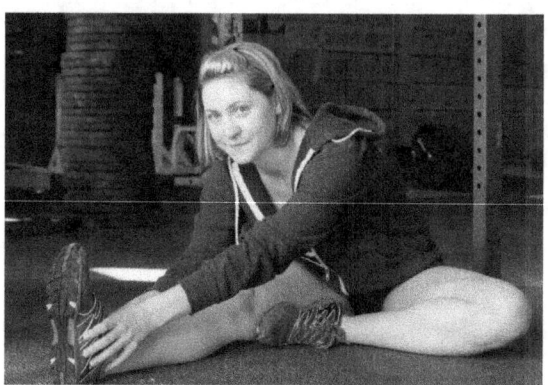

6.12   A Stretching Breakthrough

So after I had been walking for a few weeks I noticed something. In my case I had broken my left leg just below the knee. I was unable to fully extend my leg. I could get it to within about 5 degrees of being stretched straight out, but that was about it. It became too uncomfortable to try to push it any further.

The disadvantage of this situation was that every time I went to put my weight on my formally broken leg, it was already bent because I could not make it straight. I would then tend to lunge forward just a bit and ended up looking very much like an old man walking. I really had no good solution to this problem. I was trying to do my exercises and stretch my leg out, but it didn't seem to be doing the trick

My breakthrough came one day when I was down on the floor doing some push-ups. I had just completed my one and only set of push-ups and I had collapsed onto the carpet (it was only about 20 push-ups, but man did that take it out of me!) My face was buried into the carpet, I was laying on my chest, and my legs extended out behind me. Now where things get interesting is how my legs were arranged. My formally broken leg was resting knee first on the carpet. This knee was still fairly large and so it was making contact with the carpet and pushing up.

My calf and my thigh which are both connected to the knee were raised up where they connected to the knee and then they gradually came down as you moved further away from the knee. I must have laid there for about a minute and a half to two minutes. The amazing thing happened when I stood up - I was able to walk normally. My leg was fully extended and when I put my weight on my formally broken leg it was not pre-bent.

What had happened was in this face-down position, I had found a way to hyper-extend my formally broken leg. The fat knee pushing up caused the muscles, tendons, and ligaments associated with the knee area to finally stretch out to their maximum.

Now, as amazing as this breakthrough was, it didn't last forever. It seemed to last for about 10-15 minutes. However, very quickly I discovered that if I dropped to the ground and spent a minute or so in the face down position, I could recapture the benefits once again. You can imagine how happy I was when I discovered that laying on a soft bed produced most of the same benefits.

Very quickly, this new type of stretching worked its way into my daily routine. There were multiple times that my colleagues at work would pause as they passed by my office and saw me sprawled out on the floor as though I had just had a massive heart attack. I needed to quickly assure them that I was planning on going somewhere and I needed to limber up my formally broken leg before I left.

Over time I did make one more discovery involving this technique. When I laid on a bed, if I was to extend my feet over the edge of the bed, I this would maximize the slope from my raised knee to my ankle. This meant that my leg was getting the maximum stretch. No, none of this felt very comfortable, but I was willing to endure all of it because I fully believed that by stretching out the leg, the discomfort would pass and I'd be walking normally all of the time that much quicker!

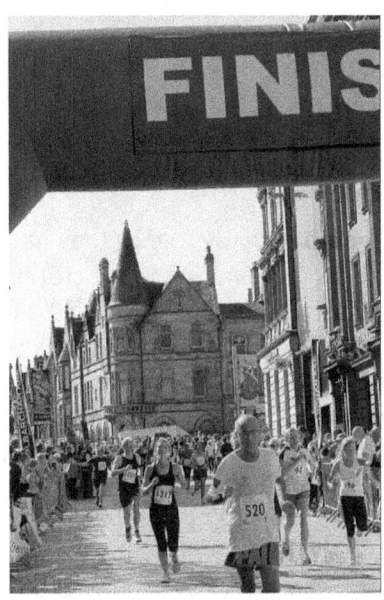

7   The Last 15%

12 months after having broken my leg, I sat down to evaluate my progress. Of course what I wanted was to put this event behind me and have everything back to where it had been before I broke my leg. However, even I in my most optimistic moments had to admit that I was not there. So where was I? By my best guess I had reached a point where I could say that I had recovered roughly 85% of the functionality with my leg that I had had before the accident.

Where were the difficulties? The first was that when I first got up in the morning, I hobbled like an old man as my formally broken leg first stretched itself out. The much more significant issue was that stairs still presented me with a significant challenge. Yes, I could climb stairs but I could feel each step. If you think about it for a moment, it makes sense. When you are climbing stairs you bend your leg and then you place your full body weight on it as you move up to the next stair. This was not comfortable!

I felt that I had stalled in my recovery. I had been walking a great deal during the past 12 months and yet I still had some significant issues that I didn't seem to be able to resolve. As I pondered these thoughts, I decided to make some changes to how I was handling my recovery.

As I had talked with my friends they had all expressed surprise when I had told them that my doctor had not signed me up for physical therapy. At the time I had understood why, but now I was having second thoughts. It took a little while, but as I thought about just exactly what people did during physical therapy I came to realize that I had the ability to create my own form of physical therapy: all I had to do was to join a gym.

So, of course, that is exactly what I ended up doing. I joined a gym in my area that charges me $20/month to belong. The first time that I went to the gym, I located one of the employees who was wearing a "trainer" shirt. I explained my "made up physical therapy" situation and asked him what would be the best way for me to exercise my formally broken leg in order to strengthen it. He then proceeded to show me three leg machines that they had at the gym.

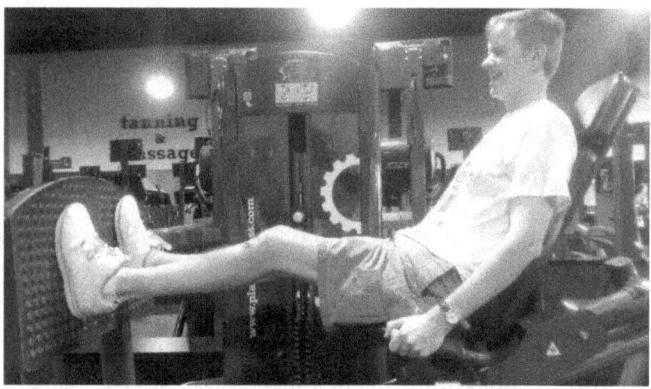

Figure 7: Seated Leg Press Exercise Machine

The first machine that I tried was called the "seated leg press". This machine allows you to set the amount of weight that you want to work with (I initially chose 30 pounds). You then position the seat so that you are sitting in a scrunched up position with your feet bent. You then extend your feet pushing up and lifting the weight that you've selected.

The trainer recommended two things. First, that I perform 15 repetitions, wait for 45 seconds, and then perform another 15 repetitions. I was ultimately to repeat my 15 repetitions four times on this machine. The trainer told me that I didn't want to hold my legs in the fully extended position. However, I did detect a slight "pop" as I reached the fully extended position so I now try to reach that position even though I don't stay there for long.

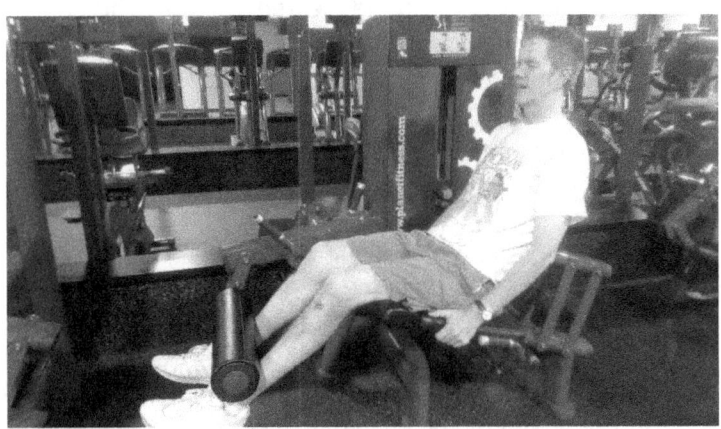

Figure 8: Leg Extension Exercise Machine

The next machine that the trainer had me try was called the "leg extension". This one consisted of me once again selecting a weight, then placing my ankles underneath a padded bar and then trying to lift the weight that I had selected. What I have discovered is that as I am working through the four sets of 15 repetitions, this machine get progressively harder. I find myself having to pause at the 10 reps mark in order to give my legs a rest before I can make it to 15 reps.

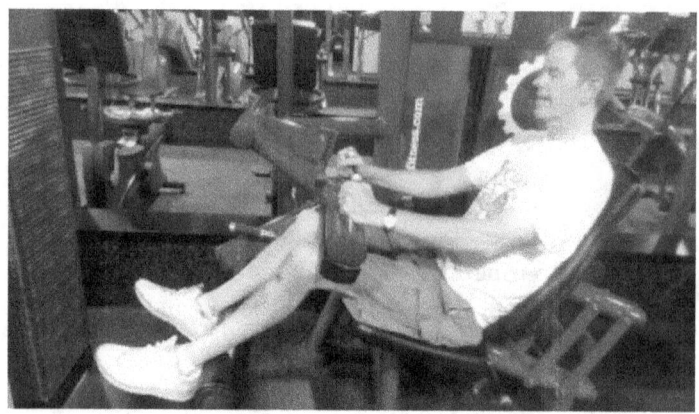
Figure 9: Seated Leg Curl Exercise Machine

The final piece of gym equipment that the trainer showed me was called the "seated leg curl". This equipment was almost the opposite of the leg extension device. I'd select my weight and then instead of trying to lift it, I would try to push a padded bar down. It took me awhile to realize it, but a critical part of this device is a bar that lays over your thighs and allows you to push against it while pushing down.

Once I had the gym membership, I started going four times a week and spending roughly 30 minutes working through these three machines. I saw an improvement in my ability to walk very quickly. I didn't see my left leg becoming any bigger to replace the fat and muscle that I had lost while it had been unused, but it did become much easier to walk.

In addition to starting to go to the gym, I got serious about my stretching exercises. Before getting out of bed each morning I would fully stretch out my formally broken leg (easy to do) to a count of 30 and then I would bend it trying to get the back of my heel to touch my butt (not so easy) for a count of 30. I would repeat both of these exercises three times before getting out of bed. None of this felt especially good, but I was determined to be able to fully stretch out my leg and this seemed to be the best way to make it happen.

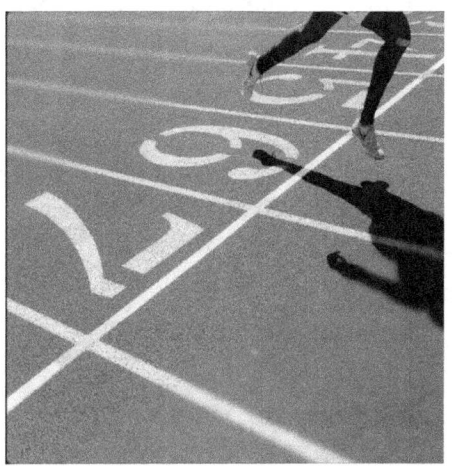

8   Conclusion

Every story has to have an ending and mine ends 15 months after my accident. Have I recovered 100% from breaking my left leg? No. Right now I would say that I am probably at about 95% of a full recovery.

Yes, sometimes when I go upstairs I can still feel my leg. However, I can now take stairs two at a time with ease. Going to the gym and exercising my leg does not feel good; however, there's a good chance that even if I had not broken my leg those types of exercises would not feel good. In the morning when I am stretching my leg out, I have an incredible range of motion but there is still more to do.

I can't actually say that I'm ever going to be able to reach 100% of a recovery. However, I am going to keep on trying. I can now walk without thinking about my formally broken leg. I sleep just fine at night and I have even been known to run quickly to catch a ball or something that has been thrown my way.

I am very pleased with my recovery; however, I've been able to reach this point because I worked very hard to get here. Just about every single day since my surgery I have been doing leg exercises, walking, or exercising at the gym. Getting better has been a part of every day.

I want you to know that you can get your old life back. However, in order to get from where you are to where you want to be is going to take a great deal of effort. It's not going to feel good and yes, there will be times that you may feel like giving up.

I'm here to urge you to keep on going. The end result when you are able to walk without a limp and without even thinking about the process of walking will be worth all of the time and effort that you have to invest in getting there. All good things take effort and it turns out that recovering from a broken leg is one of these things.

Best of luck with a speedy recovery!

Photo Credits:

Chapter 4.4 – Amazon
http://amzn.to/2esOUm5

Chapter 4.5 - WND.com
http://bit.ly/1NPpyrT

Chapter 4.6 - Simon Collison
https://www.flickr.com/photos/collylogic/

Chapter 4.7 – Kelsey
https://www.flickr.com/photos/kelseyweaverphotography/

Chapter 4.8 - Thomas Crenshaw
https://www.flickr.com/photos/tommyc/

Chapter 5 - Keith Allison
https://www.flickr.com/photos/keithallison/

Chapter 5.1 - astrid westvang
https://www.flickr.com/photos/astrid/

Chapter 5.2 - Judyth Greenburgh
https://www.flickr.com/photos/curlybird/

Chapter 5.3 - Jen Crothers
https://www.flickr.com/photos/milopup/

Chapter 6 – Islxndis
https://www.flickr.com/photos/islandis/

Chapter 6.1 - Jez Nicholson
https://www.flickr.com/photos/jnicho02/

Chapter 6.2 - Lisa Brewster
https://www.flickr.com/photos/sophistechate/

Chapter 6.3 – wackystuff
https://www.flickr.com/photos/wackystuff/

Chapter 6.4 - Bruce Aldridge
https://www.flickr.com/photos/bruce_aldridge/

Chapter 6.5 - Bev Sykes
https://www.flickr.com/photos/basykes/

Chapter 6.6 - Erica M
https://www.flickr.com/photos/swirlspice/

Chapter 6.7 - Jean KOULEV
https://www.flickr.com/photos/jean_koulev/

Chapter 6.8 - sound.photography.
https://www.flickr.com/photos/soundphotography/

Chapter 6.9 - Rev. Al Deaderick
https://www.flickr.com/photos/zsoul/

Chapter 6.10 - Thomas Hawk
https://www.flickr.com/photos/thomashawk/

Chapter 6.11 - Dan Tantrum
https://www.flickr.com/photos/tantrum_dan/

Chapter 6.12 – mgstanton
https://www.flickr.com/photos/marirn/

Chapter 7 - Paisley Scotland
https://www.flickr.com/photos/paisleyorguk/

Chapter 8 - Jeff Turner
https://www.flickr.com/photos/respres/

Other Books By
The Author

Product Management

- What Product Managers Need To Know About World-Class Product Development: How Product Managers Can Create Successful Products

- How Product Managers Can Learn To Understand Their Customers: Techniques For Product Managers To Better Understand What Their Customers Really Want

- Product Management Secrets: Techniques For Product Managers To Boost Product Sales And Increase Customer Satisfaction

- Product Development Lessons For Product Managers: How Product Managers Can Create Successful Products

- Customer Lessons For Product Managers: Techniques For Product Managers To Better Understand What Their Customers Really Want

- Product Failure Lessons For Product Managers: Examples Of Products That Have Failed For Product

Managers To Learn From

- Communication Skills For Product Managers: The Communication Skills That Product Managers Need To Know How To Use In Order To Have A Successful Product

- How To Have A Successful Product Manager Career: The Things That You Need To Be Doing TODAY In Order To Have A Successful Product Manager Career

- Product Manager Product Success: How to keep your product on track and make it become a success

Public Speaking

- Tools Speakers Need In Order To Give The Perfect Speech: What tools to use to create your next speech so that your message will be remembered forever!

- How To Create A Speech That Will Be Remembered

- Secrets To Organizing A Speech For Maximum Impact: How to put together a speech that will capture and hold your audience's attention

- How To Become A Better Speaker By Changing How You Speak: Change techniques that will transform a speech into a memorable event

- How To Give A Great Presentation: Presentation techniques that will transform a speech into a memorable event

- How To Rehearse In Order To Give The Perfect Speech: How to effectively rehearse your next speech to that your message be remembered forever!

- Secrets To Creating The Perfect Speech: How to create a speech that will make your message be remembered forever!

- Secrets To Organizing The Perfect Speech: How to organize the best speech of your life!

- Secrets To Planning The Perfect Speech: How to plan to give the best speech of your life

- How To Show What You Mean During A Presentation: How to use visual techniques to transform a speech into a memorable event

CIO Skills

- Becoming A Powerful And Effective Leader: Tips And Techniques That IT Managers Can Use In Order To Develop Leadership Skills

- CIO Secrets For Growing Innovation: Tips And Techniques For CIOs To Use In Order To Make Innovation Happen In Their IT Department

- Your Success As A CIO Depends On How Well You Communicate: Tips And Techniques For CIOs To Use In Order To Become Better Communicators

- What CIOs Need To Know About Working With Partners: Techniques For CIOs To Use In Order To Be Able To Successfully Work With Partners

- Critical CIO Management Skills: Decision Making Skills That Every CIO Needs To Have In Order To Be Able To Make The Right Choices

- How CIOs Can Make Innovation Happen: Tips And Techniques For CIOs To Use In Order To Make Innovation Happen In Their IT Department

- CIO Communication Skills Secrets: Tips And Techniques For CIOs To Use In Order To Become Better Communicators

- Managing Your CIO Career: Steps That CIOs Have To Take In Order To Have A Long And Successful Career

- CIO Business Skills: How CIOs can work effectively with the rest of the company!

IT Manager Skills

- Save Yourself, Save Your Job – How To Manage Your IT Career: Secrets That IT Managers Can Use In Order To Have A Successful Career

- Growing Your CIO Career: How CIOs Can Work With The Entire Company In Order To Be Successful

- How IT Managers Can Make Innovation Happen: Tips And Techniques For IT Managers To Use In Order To Make Innovation Happen In Their Teams

- Staffing Skills IT Managers Must Have: Tips And Techniques That IT Managers Can Use In Order To Correctly Staff Their Teams

- Secrets Of Effective Leadership For IT Managers: Tips And Techniques That IT Managers Can Use In Order To Develop Leadership Skills

- IT Manager Career Secrets: Tips And Techniques That IT Managers Can Use In Order To Have A Successful Career

- IT Manager Budgeting Skills: How IT Managers Can Request, Manage, Use, And Track Their Funding

- Secrets Of Managing Budgets: What IT Managers Need To Know In Order To Understand How Their Company Uses Money

Negotiating

- Learn How To Signal In Your Next Negotiation: How To Develop The Skill Of Effective Signaling In A Negotiation In Order To Get The Best Possible Outcome

- Learn The Skill Of Exploring In A Negotiation: How To Develop The Skill Of Exploring What Is Possible In A Negotiation In Order To Reach The Best Possible Deal

- Learn How To Argue In Your Next Negotiation: How To Develop The Skill Of Effective Arguing In A Negotiation In Order To Get The Best Possible Outcome|

- How To Open Your Next Negotiation: How To Start A Negotiation In Order To Get The Best Possible Outcome

- Preparing For Your Next Negotiation: What You Need To Do BEFORE A Negotiation Starts In Order To Get The Best Possible Deal

- Learn How To Package Trades In Your Next Negotiation

- All Good Things Come To An End: How To Close A Negotiation - How To Develop The Skill Of Closing In Order To Get The Best Possible Outcome From A Negotiation

Miscellaneous

- The Internet-Enabled Successful School District Superintendent: How To Use The Internet To Boost Parental Involvement In Your Schools

- Power Distribution Unit (PDU) Secrets: What Everyone Who Works In A Data Center Needs To Know!

- Making The Jump: How To Land Your Dream Job When You Get Out Of College!

- How To Use The Internet To Create Successful Students And Involved Parents

- How Software Defined Networking (SDN) Is Going To Change Your World Forever: The Revolution In Network Design And How It Affects You

- The Power Of Virtualization: How It Affects Memory, Servers, and Storage: The Revolution In Creating Virtual Devices And How It Affects You

Understanding how to deal with a broken leg in order to start walking again quickly

This book has been written with one goal in mind – to show you how to deal with breaking your leg. We'll cover it all: the surgery, the crutches, and the road to recovery

Let's Get You Walking Again - Fast!

What You'll Find Inside:

- **RECOVERING FROM SURGERY**

- **CRUTCHES VS WHEELCHAIR**

- **WHAT HAPPENS WHILE YOU HEAL: THE 90-DAY PLAN**

- **EMOTIONAL ISSUES**

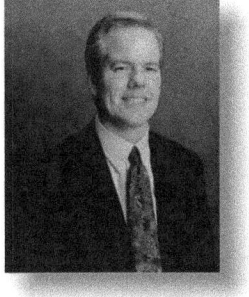

Dr. Jim Anderson brings his personal experience of dealing with a serious leg break to this book. He's lived through everything that you are going through and he asked all the right questions. Now he'll share what he learned so that your recovery can be as quick and painless as possible!

www.ingramcontent.com/pod-product-compliance
Lightning Source LLC
Chambersburg PA
CBHW070203290526
45789CB00002B/890